Essential Oils and Aromatherapy

How to Use Essential Oils for Beauty, Health, and Spirituality

Gregory Lee White

DEDICATION

For my Grandfather, W.T. White. He taught me by
example to appreciate cooking, plants, and to be
fearless when concocting new recipes and formulas.

OTHER BOOKS BY GREGORY LEE WHITE

CLUCKED – The Tale of Pickin Chicken

MAKING SOAP FROM SCRATCH: How to Make Handmade
Soap – A Beginners Guide and Beyond

CONTENTS

DISCLAIMER

The essential oil descriptions and aromatherapy
methods found in this book are not intended to
diagnose, treat, cure or prevent any illness or disease,
nor are they intended to replace proper medical help.
Essential oils are not used to "treat" medical problems.
Rather, they are meant to be used in conjunction with
modern day medicine to bring a sense of balance to the
mind, body and spirit.

LAVENDER

Lavender attracts love; ask anyone who knows plants. It whispers secrets of first kisses and sprinkles the air with luck when lovers pass by. It tells romantic tales to women who sleep beside it and sings purple lullabies that only children can hear. When the moon is full, it gives comforting advice to the daisies who know they'll be plucked petal by petal in the name of love. Lavender is humble, and bears no grudge against the roses who think they know all about human emotions. And sometimes it weeps for the lonely who have turned their backs on its magic.

-Gregory White

INTRODUCTION

Back in the 1990's, I didn't know an essential oil from a glass of orange juice. In fact, I am sure I had never even heard the term "essential oil" before I began working in the bath and body shop known as Garden Botanika. The store had a custom fragrance bar filled with fragrance oils where the customer could scent their own lotions, massage oils, and shower gels. While there were scents on the bar such as patchouli, peppermint, and lavender, they were artificial fragrances – not real essential oils from plants. But, I didn't know that. I was a newbie to the world of scent. I remember a customer asking how much an entire bottle of scent would cost (we only sold enough drops to scent their lotion) and I began spouting off how it would be very expensive since oil is extracted from plants. NOT. It was just a fake bottle of scent *called* patchouli.

A few months after the store closed, I actually learned what an essential oil was. I was embarrassed that I had given the customer bad information. When I started reading about essential oils, the massive amount of information in the books available was overwhelming. It was too much information – things a newbie just did not need to know yet, such as the in-depth (page after page) chemical composition of the oils.

I just wanted to learn which oils worked on what ailment and how to use them properly. When I set out to write this book, I remembered that experience. I decided to present a thorough book about aromatherapy and how to use essential oils, but not bog it down with technicalities that a beginner would skip over to get to the "meat and bones" of the subject.

So, this is the book I have written – how to use essential oils safely, what they are good for, how they are made, and how you can apply their use in your everyday life.

I decided to focus on the most-used essential oils. Based on my research and experience, I settled on what I consider the top fifty-five oils.

THE BACK STORY – HOW MY OWN AROMATHERAPY JOURNEY BEGAN

If someone had told me that one day I would own a bath and body company, I would not have believed them. After all, I had never even taken a chemistry class. In the big scheme of things, that did not matter because life eventually guides you in the direction it intends for you.

Back in 1998, I went to see a movie called *Practical Magic* starring Sandra Bullock and Nicole Kidman. In the film, Bullock's character Sally, a witch, opens up a little botanical shop called VERBENA. The visual of the store peaked my interest. Its harsh white walls and shelving lined with dark glass bottles; corks dipped in beeswax with unknown beauty potions lurking inside. The parchment style labels, the botanical wall hangings, a basket of bright green pears on the checkout counter; it was all eye-candy for someone who had read a lot about herbs and herbal remedies.

Shortly after that, my friend offered my previous life-partner a job as assistant manager in the Garden Botanika store she managed. The chain was in the process of closing approximately 200 stores, including hers, and her current assistant manager had already found another position. It was hard for her to find someone who only wanted to take a job for four or five months. My partner wasn't interested. I was working as an interior house painter at the time, mainly repainting vacant apartments. With flexible hours and free time, I said, "I'll do it!"

The next week I was standing behind the counter of the bath store, demonstrating hand creams and lotions, talking about soaps and body washes and helping customers blend their own fragrances in the custom fragrance bar.

Before the closing of the GB store, we began talking about starting our own bath company and began reading books of recipes and ordering in samples of fragrances. At first, like so many people, I didn't know the difference in a fragrance oil and an essential oil. Our company, Mind and Body Bath and Perfumery launched in May of 1999 selling bags of bath salt, bottles of oil burner oil and scented melt-and-pour soap. That summer, I made my first batch of handmade soap – plain, unscented. I did not use enough sodium hydroxide (lye) because the batch never really got as hard as it should have and it eventually turned rancid. So much for making soap, so we went back to the melt-and-pour.

By that autumn, it became obvious that we had different ideas about what we wanted for the Mind and Body company and decided to dissolve it, but, I was still very interested. I began searching for a new name for my own company. Having recently discovered real essential oils, I wanted something that sounded like aromatherapy. I knew that once I had learned all about them, I would eventually try to start using all natural oils in the future.

Hmm, a company owned by a guy named Gregory that sounds like the word aromatherapy? That's when I settled on Aromagregory Botanicals. In the spring of 2000, I made another batch of soap – this time using a stick blender instead of a wooden spoon and scented it with juniper breeze fragrance oil. (I hadn't gone completely natural yet.) It turned out great. Hooked,

I cleared out the last of the melt-and-pour soaps and leaned completely towards the handmade soap.

Still, sales were minimal. The manager of the apartment complex took another job and the new manager had her own painter in mind. My day job disappeared along with most of our household income. There were still a few odd painting jobs here and there but I managed to talk my way into a job with a local candle supplier. I began buying supplies from her before I ever made my first batch of soap. By the time I went to her looking for a job, I was knowledgeable about everything she sold. She taught me how to make jar candles, votives and pillars and I taught her what I knew (so far) about soap and bath products.

Summer of 2001 rolled around and I began setting up at an indoor flea market in Smyrna, TN, just outside of Nashville. My life-partner wasn't especially interested in my little company and we both knew our relationship was winding its way down. So, one weekend a month I would go by myself and set up my folding table with stacks of soap on paper doilies – scents like: gardenia, cucumber melon and blackberry sage. Of course, by this time I was also including my latest discovery – jar candles.

By that fall, I was single again, working at the candle supply company and setting up at the flea market and other outdoor festivals and events. If I remember correctly, a weekend of sales back then was around

$150. Not much. I learned Reiki (Japanese healing touch therapy) that year too. I enjoyed it but something was missing. I just didn't know what it was.

In 2003 I met Roy who was interested in the whole process of making soaps and candles (and me). When we began living together as life-partners, I wanted to reinvent the company – make it something that belonged to both of us. Roy brought something new to the table – a sense of actually building a real company around the products instead of the hobby business I had been piddling at. That is when we came up with the name The Green Pergola Soap Co. (we eventually tossed the 'the' part). What did it mean? Green was to indicate a more natural or green product. Yes, we were going green long before it was cool. Pergola is a garden arch meant to grow trailing vines. We built a pergola in the back yard and looked at it – two sides and a top, three elements, a place to grow vines. To us, the shape symbolized a place to grow the three elements of body, mind and spirit, with the use of more natural or 'green' products. During this time, Roy also learned Reiki, fulfilling a long-time interest of his in the healing arts.

Alas, we were not as green as we thought we were. During our first setup at a festival together under the name Green Pergola, our booth was set up across from another soap vendor, one with soaps only scented with real essential oils – lavenders and mints and eucalyptus and patchouli. We looked at our table of gardenia and fresh linen scented soaps and were disappointed. Out came the essential oils books that night. By the next batch, our soaps contained only real essential oils — our very first batch scented with a lavender rosemary blend.

Our repertoire of products grew and we opened our first Green Pergola store that year — a tiny 375 square foot boutique packed with soaps, candles, lotions, incense, creams and scrubs. Traffic was terrible there. Hidden by rows of trees on a stretch of road with a 55 mile per hour speed limit, people passed the store before they even knew it was there. It closed in a little under a year. We began setting up monthly at the Nashville Fairgrounds Flea Market for most of 2004 and 2005.

In 2005, we both took a long-distance course (Canadian) in aromatherapy and upon completion, became official certified aromatherapists. Official, so to speak, because the U.S. doesn't recognize the benefits of aromatherapy yet — we are a pharmacy-only dependent nation. Roy went on to advance his Reiki training and later became a licensed Reflexologist. I decided to expand my aromatherapy studies and enrolled in the 200-hour course to become a clinical certified aromatherapist, learning about anatomy and physiology and the effects of essential oils on the body. Once again, not something recognized in the U.S. In other words, if I lived in parts of Europe a doctor could refer you to me. Here, it just means I am knowledgeable about aromatherapy.

In 2006, we teamed up as "roommates" with a tea company and rented a larger store adjacent to a yoga studio. Around 675 square feet, it also came with a back office and a separate room for Reiki sessions. As roommates, we shared half the rent and half the working shift. By August 2009, the tea company pulled out of the store location and we took over the task of selling herbal teas alongside our soaps and bath products.

When the decision to incorporate came about in 2012, we decided to return to our roots and reclaim the original business name, forming Aromagregory Creative Inc. Not only the creation of our products, but also classes on soap making, a wholesale division, and books written on the subjects we had become experts in.

This is how all experts begin their journey. We take an interest in a subject and begin reading and researching. We experiment and fail. We experiment and succeed. After more than a decade of apprenticeship, we wake up one day to find we are an "expert" in the field we chose. For me, the next step was to begin teaching and writing about everything I had learned and experienced.

Gregory White

AROMATHERAPY – A BRIEF HISTORY

For centuries, people have used flowers, herbs, and roots to care for their health, their beauty, and their spirituality. The term aromatherapy evolved in the 20th century, but civilizations have been enjoying its benefits in one form or another since prehistoric times. In the earliest of times, it was the simple act of crushing plant matter. Evidence shows that cave dwellers used juniper berries as a basic antiseptic and as a food flavoring. They undoubtedly enjoyed the subtle aromatherapy value of plants through the burning of leaves and woods as well as through the sense of touch. Anyone who has ever touched a rosemary plant or peeled an orange has experienced aromatherapy.

Ancient Chinese cultures used and explored the benefits of plants and herbs. Shen Nung's classic herbal book (*Shen-nung pen ts'ao ching,* translation: *Divine Husbandman's Materia Medica*) dates back to 2,700 BC and includes 365 medicines derived from minerals, plants, and animals. Considered the father of Chinese agriculture, this legendary emperor reportedly tasted hundreds of herbs to test their medicinal value. Citrus fruit originated in China and one ancient text mentions the creation of a crude form of essential oil by means of burning the rinds in a vessel of water and collecting the floating "oils". The Chinese also used incense and burning woods in religious ceremonies.

9

Around the same time as the Chinese were exploring plants, the people of India were using aromatic plants as a vital part of their Ayurvedic medicinal system as well as for incense and spiritual practice.

The Egyptians became experts in the exotic use of aromatics. The most commonly known use is the embalming process. Cedar, sandalwood, cassia, frankincense, and myrrh, among other essential oils were blended with beeswax for that process. Most oils found in Egyptian tombs indicate they were more likely infused oils versus the pure essential oil we know today.

The science of aromatics was also for the living. These ancient Egyptians created cosmetics, perfumes and incense from fragrant plants and resins. Evidence shows that plants such as rosemary, marjoram, jasmine, chamomile, frankincense, juniper, and myrrh were in use. Most perfumes were created by blending the plant matter in oils and fats. The Egyptians became such experts in the field of aromatic cosmetics that it prompted spice trading with other countries in an effort to expand their ingredients and resources.

Pedanius Dioscorides (circa 40—90 AD) was a Greek physician, pharmacologist and botanist, and the author of *De Materia Medica,* a 5-volume encyclopedia about herbal medicine and related medicinal substances. The text was widely read for more than 1,500 years. Dioscorides began tinkering with the distilling process, but his focus was on creating floral waters, not extracting the oils from the plants.

The Persian-born physician Avicenna (980-1037 AD) is considered the inventor of distillation. Avicenna introduced the coiled cooling pipe (straight pipes were used prior to this) that allowed the condensation of steam to take place so that one could collect the evaporated oils. His efforts paved the way for the extraction of plant oils like those that we use today.

Fast forward to the 14th century. By this time, the distillation of essential oils had been around for close to two hundred years and had been highly used in pharmaceuticals for nearly a hundred years. When the Plague (a.k.a. Black Death) swept through Europe, these herbal concoctions and oils did little to help. Rumors suggest that alchemists and perfumists who worked with aromatic oils on a consistent basis avoided the disease but there is no documentation to back this up.

By the time the 16th century rolled around, perfumery had become a form of creative expression – a genuine art form. France became the capital of perfumery and its popularity demanded the farming of flowers and other precious plants. In addition, apothecary shops had become commonplace.

Throughout the 17th and 18th centuries, the perfume industry became a prosperous business across all of

Europe.

The term 'aromatherapie' was coined by a French chemist named René-Maurice Gattefossé (1881-1950) who studied the medicinal properties of essential oils for many years while working in his family's perfume business. Many aromatherapy and essential oil books report that he discovered the healing properties of lavender when a bad laboratory burn caused him to dip his arm into a vat of lavender oil. However, many feel this story has been blown out of proportion and that he was already studying the medicinal aspects of the oils when, after a burn, he decided to apply lavender oil with good results.

In the 1950's Austrian born cosmetologist Marguerite Maury introduced the idea of combining essential oils with massage and had developed some of her own massage techniques. She lectured on the concept of maintaining youth by caring and nurturing all aspects of ourselves – mind, body, and spirit. She opened aromatherapy clinics in Switzerland, England, and France, which focused mainly on the cosmetics side of essential oils, even though her passion was the therapeutic benefits of aromatherapy. Her book *The Secret of Life and Youth* was released in Britain in 1964 (released three years earlier under the title *Le Capital Jeunesse*).

In 1977, a British aromatherapist named Robert Tisserand wrote, *The Art of Aromatherapy*, the first book on aromatherapy that was written in English. It was later also published in Bulgarian, Chinese, Czech, Dutch, German, Hebrew, Italian, Japanese, Portuguese, Romanian and Spanish.

Although it has been practiced for thousands of years, Aromatherapy has only recently become popular in the Western culture. As more people learn about natural products and turn to a holistic lifestyle, they acknowledge the importance of combining the mind, body and spirit to achieve health and wellness. To this day, research is still performed to uncover all the benefits of essential oils and aromatherapy.

HOW AROMATHERAPY IS APPLIED

There are three methods for the application of aromatherapy:

- Diffusion (subtle scent in the air)

- Inhalation (breathing in essential oil vapors directly)

- Topical (applying essential oils to the skin)

DIFFUSION is the subtle use of essential oils by scenting the air with their aroma. While you do receive some of the aromatherapy benefits of breathing in the oils, the result is a mild one because the power of the oils is traveling throughout the room – not directly into your system. This method is mainly used to impart smell into a room either for cleansing the air (such as a room where someone is, or has been, ill) or for the simple pleasure of scenting the surroundings.

INHALATION is when the essential oils are breathed directly into the system. Keep in mind, essential oils are NOT inserted into the nostrils. Rather, it is as simple as breathing in the scent of the oils using nothing more than your sense of smell. I always take a cotton ball and add several drops of essential oils to it and have my client cradle the cotton ball in the palms of their hands – then bring their hands up to their nose and breathe in deeply. And I always remind them of what I mean by deep breathes, that shallow sniffs won't do – I want to see their back move up and down as they inhale. I have used this most often when a customer comes into our store with a tension headache. Just three drops of peppermint oil on the cotton ball, three deep breaths, and a ten-minute wait usually brings some relief. The inhalation method works well when seeking the emotional benefits or for immediate relief such as congestion.

TOPICAL aromatherapy is applying essentials oil directly to the skin. This can be achieved in many different ways. The most widely used method is through massage. When essential oils are used during a massage, they can be used to elevate the experience emotionally by using oils that calm and relax or with oils that are stimulating. On the other hand, the essential oils may be chosen specifically for their muscular and/or aches and pains benefits.

My own massage therapist uses both methods. Since my body is used as a tool in our business (I am constantly stirring batches of soap, lifting fifty pound buckets, and do a LOT of standing) my muscles are usually a knotted mess. When I am not manufacturing products, you will usually find me slumped over the keyboard writing or processing paperwork for orders. This is why I receive deep-tissue massages. During the massage process, she includes essential oils such as sweet marjoram for its warming effect and cypress for soothing muscular cramps. She begins the massage face-up, with the last half-hour face down. For opening up the nasal passages, she places a few drops of eucalyptus on a towel that hangs directly underneath the face cradle. On days when she knows I have been especially stressed, she may replace the eucalyptus with lavender, or even blend them together. While the latter oils mentioned are not an example of topical use, they add to the experience of the massage as a whole. The massage ends with a scalp massage with a few drops of relaxing lavender on her hands.

Another example of the topical use of essential oils is through skincare products. Lotions, creams, bath salts, soaps, and liquid soaps can all be scented with real essential oils. When these products are applied to the skin, they gradually make their way into your system. This would be especially true of lotions and creams since they are not rinsed off the body the way that soaps and body washes are. Placing a single drop of lavender essential oil on both index fingers and massaging the temples is another way to apply aromatherapy topically.

However, when including essential oils in skincare it is important to remember that less is more. Aromatherapy products are not supposed to smell as strong as the super-fragrant choices found in the big box stores and malls. If your essential oil lotion is competing with your perfume, you've probably added too much. For a full eight-ounce bottle of lotion, I usually use around fifteen drops. Half that amount would be plenty if you were using a potent oil such as pure peppermint.

PULSE POINTS – a form of topical application, scent is frequently applied to pulse points - meaning, the parts of the body where one can touch and feel the heartbeat. Perfume is usually applied at the wrists, the neck, or behind the ears – all of which are pulse points. When it comes to essential oils (versus fragrance) it is believed that application to the pulse points speeds up the absorption rate and allows the oils to work their way through the body at a faster pace. Some lesser-known pulse points are at the temples, behind the knees, the ankles, the inner elbow, and the groin area.

HOW ESSENTIAL OILS WORK

We just covered topical use of essential oils and inhalation. When you smell the aroma of essential oils, (inhalation) the scent molecules travel up the nasal passage until it reaches the olfactory bulb where it travels directly to the limbic system at the center of the brain. There, the molecules release their unique neurochemicals and cause a reaction, depending on which oil is used. Lavender brings about a sense of relaxation while peppermint perks you up. The brain knows which reaction should occur and obliges according to the essential oil.

Memory is a factor in certain parts of the limbic system. Two large limbic system structures, the amygdala and hippocampus play important roles in memory. This is why a smell will often bring back a memory. Some people will smell something and immediately think of their grandmother's house. Another scent might remind you of a vacation you took twenty years ago. It is amazing how quickly scent can trigger a memory that we thought was long forgotten.

As the molecules travel further, they interact with the lungs and respiratory system and may take different paths towards other parts of the body. Most people do not realize that a smell enters and interacts with the body. They think of smell as only happening in the room around them, a sort of "air decoration", if you will.

When applied topically (directly onto the body) essential oils are easily absorbed into your system, but more slowly than through inhalation. The use of a carrier oil to dilute the essential oils actually helps to deliver the oils across the surface of the skin, allowing them to cover a larger area than if they were applied neat (straight, no dilution).

Some people debate that the skin is a powerful barrier meant to keep out foreign substances and have stated doubt as to whether the essential oils go any further than the first few layers of skin. Yet, if this were true, the ole garlic-on-the-foot trick should not work. Peel garlic and mash is through a garlic press or chop finely, then rub it on the bottom of your foot. Within about fifteen minutes, you will actually be able to taste the garlic in your mouth. It absolutely works and, keeping this experiment in mind, it certainly sounds as if essential oils can make it through.

Another reason for topical use is to reach a specific area. For a sore muscle, it would be much better to add a little sweet marjoram and cypress to olive oil and rub it directly into the muscles versus breathing in the aroma. A drop of tea tree oil between the toes of someone with athlete's foot would certainly be more effective than taking a sniff from the bottle.

When using essential oils for aromatherapy, the method in which you use them depends entirely on the physical condition or state of mind you are trying to overcome.

- For a stomachache blend 2 drops of peppermint in teaspoon of carrier oil and massage on abdomen

- When stressed, place one drop of lavender oil on your index finger, rub your two index fingers together, and then massage your temples.

- Long study night and need to pass a test? Rub a little basil and clove on your pencil. The scent and your handling of the pencil will improve concentration and memory retention.

- Too many mosquitoes in the yard? Lemon Eucalyptus and Citronella blended in a little alcohol and water makes and excellent natural insect repellent spray. (Shake before each use).

- For grief, place a few drops of geranium oil on a handkerchief and take it with you to a funeral.

- To relieve the pain of a simple toothache when you can't get to the dentist, use one drop of clove oil on your fingertip and massage the gum around the offending tooth.

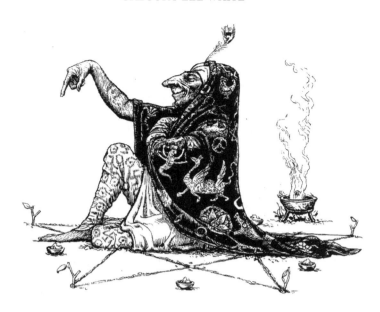

HOW ESSENTIAL OILS ARE MADE

DISTILLATION

Many of the most common essential oils are steam distilled. It is the same process you see in the movies of people making moonshine. Sometimes the big copper coil and all are used. The plant matter, which may consist of flowers, roots, leaves, and more, is placed in the distillation apparatus with water (also known as an alembic vessel or simply a "still") where the water and plant matter are heated. The plant material releases aromatic material as the steam forces the essential oils in the plants to burst open and escape, evaporating into the steam. The temperature of the steam is carefully controlled - just enough to force the plant material to let go of the essential oil, yet not so hot it would burn the plant material or the essential oil.

The steam containing the essential oils passes through a cooling chamber, causing condensation. The collecting tube is often coiled and is housed within an outer container through which the cool water flows. This allows the fluid to condense and drip into the collector. In the collector, the essential oil separates from the hydrosol or aqueous portion. Distillation may take anywhere from a couple of hours to nearly twenty hours, depending on the plant matter being distilled.

This is where hydrosols come from. They are literally the water used in the distillation process.

EXPRESSION

This is also known as cold pressing. Most citrus peel oils are expressed mechanically, or cold pressed (similar to olive oil extraction). Due to the relatively large quantities of oil in citrus peel and low cost to grow and harvest raw materials, citrus-fruit oils are cheaper than most other essential oils. You can actually squeeze essential oil out when you peel an orange or a lemon. No heat source is needed for this extraction method, which is why it is called "cold pressing." While today large machines do all the pressing, in early times the rinds were hand squeezed onto sponges in order to collect the precious oils.

ENFLEURAGE

This is an older method not frequently used today. In cold enfleurage, a large framed plate of glass, called a chassis, smeared with a layer of animal fat (usually lard or tallow) is allowed to set. Most oils collected with this method are flowers. Petals or whole flowers placed on the fat diffuse their scent into the fat over the course of 1-3 days. The spent flowers are replaced with fresh ones until the fat has reached a desired degree of fragrance. This procedure was developed in southern France in the 19th century for the production of high-grade concentrates. In hot enfleurage, solid fats are heated and botanical matter stirred into the fat. Spent botanicals are repeatedly strained from the fat and replaced with fresh material until the fat is saturated with fragrance. This method is the oldest known procedure for preserving plant fragrance substances. Jasmine was commonly a popular flower that went through the enfleurage process.

SOLVENT EXTRACTED

Solvent extracted is almost exactly how it sounds. This is how *absolutes* are made. Flowers are covered with a solvent (hexane, for example) which extracts the essential oil from the flowers/plants. Solvent extraction does not always have to mean the solvent was unnatural. Sometimes solid oils, fats, or carbon dioxide are used (think high-tech-enfleurage). The primary reason for using this method is for flowers that are too delicate to be steam distilled. Jasmine Absolute is made using the solvent extraction method.

INFUSED OIL

There have been many times over the years that I have encountered people that tell me they make their own essential oils. I immediately ask them if they own a farm, because distilling essential oils takes an enormous amount of plant matter. When the answer is no, I ask them about the process – only to find that they are actually making infused oils. I can remember back many years ago when I tried this and thought I was making my own essential oils. I took the peel of several oranges and packed a canning jar full then poured sweet almond oil over the peels, capped it, and allowed it to sit for two weeks. The result was sweet, orange-smelling oil. However, when I purchased my first essential oil book some weeks later I discovered that my jar of citrusy oil was far from being an actual essential oil. This is how we learn: experimentation and research.

Infused oils involve taking plants and allowing them to soak in carrier oil, usually a liquid vegetable oil, for an extended period, giving the plant time to release its properties into the base. Most of the time, the method is to leave the jar sitting in the sunlight (such as a windowsill) so that the carrier oil will be heated gently and naturally, which encourages the plant matter to release more of its precious oils.

While it may not be an essential oil, this is still an excellent way to make your own herbal-based massage oils. The key to success is absolutely cleanliness. The jars should first be sterilized (a dishwasher will do) then thoroughly dried. There should be absolutely no water, not even a drop, left inside your glass jar because water will be the foundation for the growth of bacteria.

If using fresh herbs from your garden, wash them to get rid of any dirt or bugs, and allow them to dry completely. I don't mean turning them into a dried herb – just the process of getting all water off of the plant. If this means putting your project off until the next day, so be it. Knowing this, you may want to cut your plants and rinse them the day before you plan your infusion project. You can speed up the process by blotting the plants with paper towels.

When your plants/herbs are completely dry, you want to bruise them – meaning, you're going to pinch or rub the leaves slightly to help bring some of the essential oils out. Some people go a step further and chop the herbs. Then, pack your jar at least half-way with the herb (almost all the way to the top is best) and cover with your carrier oil. Fill the jar with oil as far as you can. Leaving a lot of airspace at the top gives more chance for mold to occur.

Olive oil is a popular choice but many people also choose: canola oil, sunflower oil, safflower oil, or even common vegetable oil. You may also use more exotic oils, such as sweet almond or grapeseed oil. Just be sure not to choose oils that become rancid easily, especially if you are going to place your infusion in a sunny windowsill.

Cap the jar tightly and gently shake or swirl the contents each day.

I never use the sunlight method when I infuse oils. I prefer to place the jars in a dark, room-temperature spot for about two weeks. There are many who feel that the addition of sunlight does more harm than good to the integrity of your base oil. Furthermore, the sunlight and heat can cause condensation in the jar. Usually, the darkroom method will give you a lighter colored finished product.

After the herbs have steeped for a few weeks, strain the contents through cheesecloth several times so that no plant matter remains in the carrier oil. Bottle and store away from light. The product should be good for at least six months, although I have seen some infused oils last for a couple of years. At this point, you may also choose to add vitamin E to the oil by breaking open several capsules and spilling their contents into your infused oil, which will help with rancidity. If you have chosen oils that tend to go rancid more quickly than others do, you may choose to store your finished product in the refrigerator.

ESSENTIAL OIL YIELD – HOW MUCH IS ACTUALLY IN THAT LITTLE BOTTLE

The primary reason for price fluctuation with essential oils is that the raw plant matter has different yields. The yield is measured by how much essential oil is obtained, on average, from a specific amount of planted crop (such as an acre).

An acre of orange trees would yield pounds and pounds more essential oil than an acre planted in lemon balm (Melissa), because oranges contain a large amount of oil in their peel. Lemon balm, on the other hand, is a plant that has high water content but a low amount of essential oil. Its yield per acre would be much lower. This is why Melissa oil costs approximately 100 times more than orange oil. This is an example of two vastly different plant yields. Many plants have similar oil content but not the same. In addition, conditions such as soil quality and weather will affect the yield of a crop from year to year.

Let's take lavender as an example so that we can break down the numbers even further. Before moving onto to the lavender essential oil numbers, let's talk about dried lavender so that you have a frame of reference for both. According to a report done by Washington State University (Washington is the number one grower of lavender in the United States) "an acre of Healthy, mature Lavandin Grosso plants should yield between 4 and 6 bundles per plant (bundles averaging about 150 stems per bundle). Assuming an average of 5 bundles per plant, and assuming a planting density of 2,400 plants per acre, a well-managed acre of Grosso should yield approximately 12,000 bundles. It takes between 12 and 15 dried bundles of Grosso to yield a pound of dried lavender buds. Another way to look at yield of dried buds is that one Grosso plant should yield between ¼ and ½ lb of dried buds. This equates to a little over 1,000 lbs of dried Grosso lavender buds per acre."

Just a note: lavandin is a hybrid – a cross between true lavender and spike lavender.

Now, let's see how much oil we can get from an acre of lavender. The above example is for a lavandin grosso, which usually yields twice as much oil as regular lavenders. The plants also grow larger which is why there are fewer planted per acre. That being said, since regular lavender is mainly what is used in aromatherapy, I'd like to focus on two varieties that yield approximately the same amount of oil – Provence and English.

According to another study done in Washington State, these two true lavenders yield about 25 pounds of oil per acre during a good crop year. This is at the high end of the spectrum, with 12 pounds being in the low range. However, for our purposes, let's use the 25 pound figure. This weight is based on plants that are full-grown. Full-grown English lavender can be about 2 to 3 feet tall and approximately twice as wide. An acre of English lavender will hold around 2900 plants.

2900 plants divided by 25 equals 116. It takes 116 plants to make one pound of lavender essential oil. Most essential oils are sold in ½ ounce (15ml) bottles. There are 16 ounces in a pound. You can use a pound of oil to fill 32 of those ½ ounce bottles. So, 116 divided by 32 equals 3.625 plants. Rounding down to 3.5 to keep it simple, that means, inside each ½ ounce bottle of English lavender essential oil there are 3.5 lavender bushes that were originally 2 to 3 feet tall and 4 to 6 feet wide.

Can you image throwing three or four of these lavender bushes into your bathtub? For one thing, they wouldn't fit. This is precisely why only a few drops of essential oil are needed whether it is for a bath, massage oil, or a small jar of cream. Most people don't realize how potent essential oils really are. I hope that the above math demonstrates the strength of pure essential oils. A few drops are all you need. Period.

UNDERSTANDING NOTES – TOP, MIDDLE, AND BASE

'Notes' is a term used in perfumery to describe the category a scent falls into, based on its scent and staying power. Essential oil was perfume for centuries before the invention of artificial fragrance so they are assigned notes that describe where they fall on the perfumer's scale. The three types of fragrance notes are as follows: top notes, also known as head notes; middle notes, also known as heart notes; and base notes. Understanding these notes is essential to creating the perfect blend of oils – especially when it comes to perfume and fragrance.

TOP NOTES are first impression scents, the one that you smell first when you breathe in a blend. Top notes have tiny, light molecules that evaporate quickly. These top note scents are often described as cheerful, bright, light, refreshing. Citrus oils fall into the category of top notes.

MIDDLE NOTES are scents that emerge from a blend right after the top notes have evaporated away and give perfumes their main body, their "heart," which is why the middle note is sometimes called the 'heart note.' Middle notes do not evaporate as quickly as top notes and linger on the skin longer. Lavender is an example of a middle note.

BASE NOTES describe the oils that stay with you the longest. They have heavy molecules that take much longer to evaporate. Base notes add depth and richness to a blend as well as acting as an anchor for the entire perfume. Sandalwood and Patchouli are both examples of base notes. In perfume, you smell these scents after the tops and middles have faded away and the entire blend has settled in on the skin.

This is why one should always wait thirty minutes or more before they make a final decision about choosing a new perfume. The scent you spray on in the first few minutes will not be the same one you smell a half hour later.

Let's go through a practical example. Lay out three cotton balls on the kitchen counter. On the first, place a drop of sweet orange oil (a top note); on the second, a single drop of lavender oil (middle note); on the third, a single drop of sandalwood oil (base note). Immediately you smell all three very clearly because they are fresh out of the bottle, but oxygen and the evaporation process are about to change that. Leave the house to do some errands and when you come back after a couple of hours, you notice that you can barely smell the orange oil (the top note and its tiny molecules are quickly floating away). But, the lavender and the sandalwood cotton balls are still nice. Fast forward to that evening at bedtime – you can still smell the lavender but it is no longer as strong (the middle note's slightly larger molecules are fighting to hang around). Sandalwood still smells good. By the next morning the orange has completely disappeared, the lavender is barely hanging on, and the sandalwood is still going strong (the base oil's heavy molecules are thick and lazy, hanging onto the cotton ball and yawning – you might not get rid of them for a few days). This, in a nutshell, is how 'notes' work.

The notes listed in the following chart are the 55

essential oils this book focuses on. It is not a complete list of all essential oils and their notes.

TOP NOTES:	MIDDLE NOTES:	BASE NOTES:
Anise	Allspice	Amyris
Basil	Cajeput	Angelica Root
Bergamot	Camphor, White	Cedarwood Atlas
Citronella	Cardamom	Clove Bud
Eucalyptus	Carrot Seed	Frankincense
Galbanum	Chamomile, German	Ginger *middle/base*
Grapefruit	Chamomile, Roman	Helichrysum
Lemon	Cinnamon Leaf	Myrrh
Lemongrass	Clary Sage	Patchouli
Lime	Coriander	Sandalwood
Litsea *top/middle*	Cypress	Ylang Ylang
Mandarin	Eucalyptus, Lemon	*middle/base*
Melissa	Geranium	
top/middle	Ginger *middle/base*	
Orange, Sweet	Jasmine Absolute	
Peppermint	Juniper Berry	
Petitgrain	Lavender	
Ravensara	Litsea *top/middle*	
Spearmint	Marjoram	
Tangerine	Melissa *top/middle*	
	Neroli	
	Nutmeg	
	Palmarosa	
	Pepper, Black	
	Pine	
	Rose	
	Rosemary	
	Tea Tree	
	Ylang Ylang	
	middle/base	

CARRIER OILS

Carrier oils come from the seeds, kernels, and flesh from a wide variety of plants. Since many essential oils are not for application directly on the skin, carrier oils are the vessel that delivers the properties of the essential oils over the surface of the skin. The essential oil is eventually absorbed into the body. When you mix essential oils with carrier oils, you not only get the aromatherapy benefits of the EO's but also the vitamins and individual properties of the carrier oil used.

Another word for carrier oil is *base oil*. Unlike essential oils, they actually *are* oily to the touch because they are comprised of essential fatty acids. When a customer looks confused as to what I mean when I talk about carrier oils, I simply use the term *vegetable oil* and this bring a look of ah-ha-I-understand to their face. I go on to explain the different types of carrier oils, how their quality differs from a bottle of vegetable oil found in the grocery, although many good carriers are available at the supermarket.

Below is a listing of some of the most common carrier oils used in creating aromatherapy and massage blends. While it may not be a complete list of every carrier oil available, it represents the best-known and most readily available oils. A good ratio for blending essential oils into carrier oil is approximately 10 to 15 drops of essential oil blended in 1 ounce (30 ml) of carrier oil.

Sweet Almond Oil *(Prunus dulcis)* is a great moisturizer and helps condition the skin. It also helps balance the skin as far as moisture loss and has a positive effect for itchy skin. It is a frequent choice for massage blends because it does not penetrate the skin too quickly and stays on the surface longer than other oils without being greasy. Obtained from the dried kernels of the almond tree, be sure to steer clear if you are allergic to almonds.

Apricot Kernel Oil *(Prunus armeniaca)* is also a good moisturizer and helps condition the skin. A little greasier than almond oil, it makes a good addition to a massage blend because it spreads so easily. It is particularly helpful for dehydrated, delicate, mature, and sensitive skin, and it helps to sooth inflammation.

Avocado Oil *(Persea Americana)* is a great moisturizer and often used for creating aromatherapy massage blends. Avocado oil contains vitamins A, D, and E, which makes it healing as well as moisturizing. Try to buy the dark green avocado oil – the darker the better. Lighter avocado oils usually have been bleached. Avocado oil is excellent for people suffering from eczema or psoriasis, and is useful when treating dehydrated, undernourished, sun-damaged skin as it potentially helps with regenerating the skin and softening the tissue.

Canola Oil *(Brassica napus L or Brassica campestris L.*

or *Brassica Rapa var.)* was formerly known as rapeseed oil and is a good moisturizer but is less saturated than other fats. It is not usually the first choice when creating luxury blends; it is a good carrier oil to use in a pinch since many people already have it in their kitchen cabinets. It has a greasy texture and is slow to absorb.

Cocoa butter *(Theobroma cacao)* is used to lay down a protective layer that holds the moisture to the skin, so it is an excellent skin softener. It has a natural chocolate scent but it is also available in unscented versions and is frequently recommended for the prevention of stretch marks in pregnant women, as well as a treatment for chapped skin and lips, and as a daily moisturizer to prevent dry, itchy skin. It is also helpful with scars; however, cocoa butter is extremely hard. So, if you are making a salve or balm, it needs to be melted and blended with a softer oil so that it becomes workable.

Coconut Oil Fractionated *(Cocos nucifera)* has become my new favorite carrier oil. It absorbs into the skin quickly and has an indefinite shelf life. Fractionated coconut oil is processed in a way that removes all the long chain fatty acids, leaving only the healthy medium chain fatty acids. Due to the way it is processed, fractionated coconut oil has a high concentration of Capric acid and Caprylic acid, which gives it an amazing amount of antioxidant and disinfecting properties. Regular coconut oil is solid at room temperature and has a greasy feeling when applied to the skin.

Grapeseed Oil *(Vitus vinifera)* is a lightweight oil that absorbs into the skin quickly without leaving a heavy greasy feeling. Unlike most other carrier oils, grapeseed is not cold-pressed but solvent extracted, so trace amounts of the solvent could possibly be left behind. While others report that it has a shelf life between six months to a year, I've never found this to be true in my own experience. It seemed to only last three to four months before going rancid after opening the bottle. Best if stored in refrigerator to lengthen the shelf life.

Hazelnut Oil *(Vitus vinifera)* is low in saturated fatty acids, and is reported to help tighten the skin. Especially useful for clients with oily skin, despite the fact that it leaves an oily film on the surface of the skin. It is a good toner and aids in the regeneration of cells and strengthening of capillaries. With astringent properties, hazelnut would make a good base for blends meant to treat acne.

Jojoba *(Simmondsia chinensis)* is an excellent emollient for skin conditions like psoriasis, because it has a chemical composition very close to the skin's own sebum. It is suitable for all skin types, beneficial for spotty and acne conditions, and good for sensitive and oily skin. Jojoba is actually not oil at all but rather, a liquid wax. When added to other oils at 10% ratio, it helps to prevent other oils from going rancid and lengthens their shelf life.

Kukui Nut Oil *(Aleurites moluccans)* also known as Candlenut oil, is native to Hawaii and is high in linoleic acid. It is quickly absorbed into the skin and is excellent for skin conditioning after sun exposure, as well as for acne, eczema, and psoriasis. It offers just the right amount of lubrication without leaving a greasy feeling. It has been used to treat burns and wounds as well as a scalp and hair conditioner.

Olive Oil (Olea europaea) is one of the heavier carriers and tends to leave an oily feeling on the skin. Olive oil is known to be good for burns, inflammation, and arthritis. While it isn't the preferred oil used in aromatherapy, it is often used as part of a blend of carrier oils. Mediterranean women have used it for centuries as a "wrinkle cream" around the edges of the eyes.

Shea butter *(Butyrospermum parkii)* comes two different ways – in its natural state and refined. Natural shea butter is yellow in color and has a nutty scent to it. Refined shea butter has undergone a cleaning process so it is white and odorless. Which one you decide to use depends totally on personal preference. Shea butter is thought to be an effective treatment for the following conditions: fading scars, eczema, rashes, burns, dry skin, dark spots, skin discolorations, chapped lips, stretch marks, wrinkles, and in soothing the irritation of psoriasis. While it isn't actually considered a carrier oil, shea butter is still soft enough to use in aromatherapy work.

Sunflower Oil *(Helianthus annuus)* is a less expensive alternative to olive oil. It contains Vitamin E, so it naturally resists going rancid. It penetrates the skin well and doesn't leave behind an oily residue. Sunflower oil is reported to be beneficial for the treatment of bruises and other skin diseases. Sunflower oil, like other oils, can retain moisture in the skin.

CREATING ESSENTIAL OIL BLENDS

The most important part of creating the perfect essential oil blend is: 1. Have a clear focus on what you want to accomplish. 2. Be knowledgeable about essential oils and their benefits. 3. Use only pure essential oils.

Generally, essential oil blends are created for either an aesthetic or a therapeutic purpose.

THE AESTHETIC BLEND

An aesthetic essential oil blend is all about beauty and scent and has very little to do with the healing properties of the oils. However, some may feel that blends created totally for emotional purposes may fall into the aesthetic category. For example, I created a meditation blend that contains: sandalwood, cedarwood, frankincense, myrrh, and clove. It is a blend heavy on the base oils that have been used for centuries for meditation. The addition of the clove was my own choice to give it a spicy undertone, but had nothing to do with the properties of clove.

Another example is two lavender soaps we make: lavender orange and lavender lime. The lavender orange blend was made as a children's soap because the two mixed together smell surprisingly like Fruit Loops cereal (I have no idea why, but they do). The Lavender Lime soap was created as a gateway soap to get men to try lavender. If you ask, most men will say that lavender is a "girl scent." Add the crisp, citrusy-green lime scent and the smell changed into something men like. Both of these essential oil blends were created solely for the smell, nothing more – the benefits of relaxing lavender just happen to be a bonus.

Creating blends for perfumes or to scent the home are examples of using essential oils for aesthetic reasons.

THE THERAPEUTIC BLEND

When you create a therapeutic aromatherapy blend for someone else, you need to do a lot of detective work. If it is for yourself, you should already know all the answers, but perhaps no one ever taught you which questions to ask. A therapeutic blend should be multipurpose and go after more than one condition or discomfort.

Top and middle notes are most often used for acute conditions while middle and base notes go after the chronic conditions. This is because base notes with their heavier molecules stay in the system longer.

ESSENTIAL OILS AND AROMATHERAPY

Also, base note oils can act as a fixative for the lighter top and middle notes, giving them more staying power – a perfect example as to why a good and balanced blend should contain all the notes.

So, what is the difference in an acute and a chronic condition?

An *Acute condition* is usually a short-lived one such as stress over a recent event, a cold or the flu, anxiety over having to give a speech, or sleeplessness that popped up out of nowhere and hasn't been going on that long.

A *Chronic condition* is one that is more long-term. Perhaps someone has had insomnia for over four months or they have been getting headaches for most of their adult life.   Chronic may also mean something more serious such as having HIV, Diabetes, or even asthma.

Aromatherapy is often used for both acute and chronic conditions. <u>But, as with any illness or disease, you should still consult a medical doctor. Aromatherapy is NOT a replacement for medical attention and supervision.</u>

The following is a fictitious case study on Jane Smith, to create an aromatherapy blend for her to use.

Jane has two acute conditions (stress and infrequent migraines) and one chronic condition (endometriosis).

First, we will ask her a few questions, including: sleep patterns, allergies, last visit to doctor, whether or not she is pregnant, if she has a healthy diet, etc. The reason these questions are asked is not to make a diagnosis (which only a doctor should do) but to give an aromatherapist a full picture of the client's health and lifestyle.

People don't always associate everyday habits with their discomforts. When you ask someone to write down what they are eating, how well they sleep, their digestion, etc. – it puts a lifestyle history right in front of them and it forces them to think about it. If someone is telling you they are not eating well, they don't sleep, they are getting headaches, and they haven't been to the doctor in over two years, it could be a good time to nudge them with a little friendly advice about scheduling a checkup with their medical doctor.

Other questions help you create the perfect blend. In our sample case study, we learn that the subject is allergic to peanuts so we definitely know we will NOT be blending her essential oils into a base of peanut oil. Pregnancy is another important question since certain essential oils are best avoided during pregnancy. If the person has high or low blood pressure, there are other oils to avoid.

These are *contraindications*. (For more information, see the section on Safety)

Asking the client about their essential oil likes and dislikes is another important question. In our example, clary sage makes Jane nauseous. While it may appear in the choices of oils that are good for her conditions, she is certainly not going to continue to use the blend if it makes her sick to her stomach.

Next, we are going to research and list the oils for each condition. When you have finished with all conditions, there should be a pattern of repetition. In the Jane Smith case study example, we find that chamomile appears in her first and second condition, so we cross out chamomile in the second condition and place the number '2' beside chamomile in the first list. We also find chamomile again for her third condition. Cross it out in the 3rd list and place a '3' beside chamomile in the first list. This provides a quick reference as to which oils appear several times. Simply circling oils on a large list can end up looking messy and cause confusion.

Under ideal circumstances, a base note will appear in the list for the chronic condition. However, in this case (endometriosis) no base notes are suggested, so we proceed with whichever oils appear the most times in all conditions.

For our essential oil blend, we select Lavender and Chamomile because they appeared in all three of her conditions – the two acute conditions and the one chronic. We select Marjoram as it appeared in both her first and second conditions. Omit Clary sage, even though it appeared in both her first and second conditions, because of Jane's nauseous reaction to it.

From there we create our essential oil blend and mix it in a carrier base: Essential Oils Chosen: 3 drops chamomile, 3 drops marjoram, 6 drops lavender mixed into a one ounce (30 ml) carrier oil blend containing – half ounce olive oil and half ounce jojoba. (The carrier oil blend was just a personal preference.) More lavender was used because it is generally tolerated in higher amounts by most people and is good for almost every ailment.

(case study begins next page. I have selected a different font so that you can easily see how a case study form looks).

ESSENTIAL OILS AND AROMATHERAPY

Main Condition: **ACUTE STRESS**

TOP	MIDDLE	BASE
Lime	Chamomile-2,3	
Mandarin	Cinnamon	
Orange	Geranium	
Petigrain	Juniper	
Bergamot	Lavender-2,3	
Clary Sage-2	Marjoram-2	
Grapefruit	Melissa	
Lemon	Palmarosa	
	Peppermint	
	Pine	
	Rosemary	

Secondary Condition: **ACUTE MIGRAINES**

TOP	MIDDLE	BASE
~~Clary Sage~~	~~Chamomile~~	
	~~Lavender~~	
	~~Marjoram~~	

Third Condition: **CHRONIC ENDOMETRIOSIS**

TOP	MIDDLE	BASE
	~~Chamomile~~	
	~~Lavender~~	

SAMPLE QUESTIONNAIRE

Client's Name in full: Jane Smith
Occupation: homemaker, volunteer committees
Active or Inactive: active
Medical History: diagnosed with endometriosis in June, 2010. Otherwise, has been completely healthy. Has no children, no plans for children.
Medication: naproxen
Hospitalization: outpatient Laparoscopy, October 2011
Last visit/s to Doctor: January 2013
Vitamins: multivitamin, green tea extract pills, fish oil pills
Allergies: peanuts

Headaches: migraines every 8 – 10 weeks, mild to severe.
Sleep: Bedtime is 11:00 pm, wakes at 6:00 am. Wakes feeling rested, except for the day after a migraine.
Bowel: regular, daily mornings
Digest   4 main groups Y or N – eats a balanced diet, 5 light meals per day.
Reproductive Pregnant Y or N - No
General Health: good
Energy Level   High or Low: high, 90% of the time.
Pre-existing Conditions: *endometriosis, no other*
Stress Level – High Medium Low: MEDIUM

Notes: Jane says she has taken on too many projects involving church functions, charities and school projects and needs to cut back. Usually, when she is under deadlines for these events is when her migraines occur. Says her stress is from overextending herself and when she is not involved in so many projects, she has virtually no stress.

Likes/dislikes of Eos. Dislike of clary sage. Jane states that she tried clary sage in the past and the scent makes her extremely nauseous.

Essential Oils Chosen: 3 drops chamomile, 3 drops marjoram, 6 drops lavender

Carrier Oil Added: 30 mls – 15 olive oil, 15 jojoba

Home Treatment Remarks: massage on back of neck in the evenings before bed. When a migraine is coming, rub on back of neck and at temples.

ADDITIONAL NOTES: Suggested that Jane think about which committees were the most important to her and to think about possibly taking on less responsibility with the others.

The above therapeutic example of a case study is a detailed version of how an aromatherapist might go about creating an essential oil blend for a client. You can still create a blend for therapeutic purposes without going into that much detail by learning your oils and their properties and by remembering to use only a few oils in a blend.

SAFETY GUIDELINES – USING ESSENTIAL OILS SAFELY

With a few exceptions, most essential oils are perfectly safe if used correctly. In aromatherapy, remember the term **less is more** because it is rare that more than a few drops of any essential oil are needed at any given time.

First, never use essential oils undiluted on the skin. There are instances when a qualified aromatherapist will suggest that an essential oil be used neat (undiluted) but until you have done a large body of research on essential oils and aromatherapy, stay safe and always dilute your oils. Dilution doesn't have to always mean a carrier oil. Essential oils can be diluted in: lotions, creams, shampoo, bath oil, bath salts, pure alcohol (to make perfume), body scrubs, and even room and body sprays.

Some essential oils are simply too toxic and should not be used in aromatherapy. These oils include: bitter almond, buchu, camphor (brown or yellow), sassafras, calamus, horseradish, mugwort, mustard, pennyroyal, rue, savory, southernwood, tansy, thuja, wintergreen, wormseed and wormwood. Do not consider the above a complete list. Just because an oil is not listed above does not mean it is safe. Always research all essential oils before use.

OILS TO AVOID DURING PREGNANCY

Bitter almond, basil, clary sage, clove bud, hyssop, sweet fennel, juniper berry, marjoram, myrrh, peppermint, rose, rosemary, sage, thyme and wintergreen.

PHOTOSENSITIVITY.

Some essential oils are photosensitive, which means they can make you sensitive to sunlight. When these oils are applied to the skin they can cause a rash or burn when exposed to sunlight. After using these oils, it is recommended that you stay out of the sun (or tanning bed) for a couple of days. You will find that many of the citrus oils fall into this category. Some of the photosensitive essential oils are: grapefruit, orange, tangerine, mandarin, lemon, and bergamot, but again, this is not a comprehensive list as individuals can sometimes exhibit photosensitivity to substances which are not known to invoke that response.

CONTRAINDICATIONS

Contraindications are the "warning labels" of essential oils and let you know which oils you should avoid if you have certain medical conditions such as: asthma, high blood pressure, low blood pressure, diabetes, pregnancy, etc. It cannot be said enough – research your essential oils before use, especially if you have a pre-existing condition.

PERFORMING A PATCH TEST

Before using a new essential oil, it is advisable to perform a skin patch test. You can test your skin's reaction by dabbing a small amount on the inside of your arm. If you notice any redness, burning or irritation, discontinue using the oil immediately and wash the area thoroughly with plain soap and water.

INGESTING ESSENTIAL OILS

I must come out as saying that I do not promote the internal use of essential oils, and there are some essential oils that should never be orally consumed under any circumstances. (Please see section on ingesting essential oils – the big debate) The main problem is that there are unqualified and untrained people promoting internal use. Always seek out a trained aromatherapist or holistic doctor before considering this option – a well-delivered sales pitch is not the same as consulting a qualified practitioner!

THE CHEMICAL CONSTITUENTS OF ESSENTIAL OILS

Essential oils can be subdivided into two distinct groups of chemical constituents; the hydrocarbons which are made up almost exclusively of terpenes (monoterpenes, sesquiterpenes, and diterpenes), and the oxygenated compounds which are primarily esters, aldehydes, ketones, alcohols, phenols, and oxides.

TERPENES - Terpenes and terpenoids are the primary constituents of the essential oils of many types of plants and flowers. In others words, they are the building blocks of essential oils. There are two classes of terpenes: *monoterpenes* and *sesquiterpenes*. For a variety of industrial reasons, some perfumery companies "deterpenize" oils (lemon, for example where they remove the d-limonene) for the sake of creating a stronger scent. However, when you remove the terpenes, you also remove the main healing properties of these oils.

ESTERS - Esters are the result of a chemical reaction between organic acids and alcohols or phenols, and are the most widespread group found in essential oils. Most are generally mild and very stable compounds and their scents usually have a somewhat fruity tone to them, while others can be medicinal and potent. Esters are effective on inflammations and skin irritations, are anti-fungal, and have a relaxing and calming effect on the nervous system.

ALDEHYDES – aldehydes are most often found in lemony-smelling essential oils such as: citronella, lemongrass, and lemon eucalyptus but some oils have herbaceous and sometimes dry scents. Citrals are widely used in perfumery (synthetic aldehydes played an important role in the creation of Channel No 5). They are sometimes irritating to the skin and should be diluted before use, but they are highly effective when their scent is inhaled. Aldehydes have anti-infectious, anti-viral, anti-inflammatory and calming properties.

KETONES – when used responsibly, ketones can have powerful benefits including the ability to: calm, sedate, heal wounds, work as an expectorant, and be used as an anti-inflammatory. But, they can also be the most potentially dangerous when safety guidelines are ignored. The most toxic ketone is Thujone found in mugwort, sage, tansy, thuja and wormwood oils. Other toxic ketones found in essential oils are pulegone in pennyroyal, and pinocamphone in hyssop. It is said that ketones can cause epileptic seizures, induce abortion and wreak havoc on the central nervous system. Misuse usually occurs when proper daily dosages are ignored, resulting in a toxic buildup in the body. For example, let's say that an oil has a daily recommended dosage of only four drops on the skin and every day you have been using six drops. The theory is that those extra two drops cannot escape your system and will build up over time – so, after ten days, you have an extra twenty drops roaming around your system. Oils that contain a smaller amount of ketones include: roman chamomile, lavandin, peppermint, and spearmint.

ALCOHOLS - are known for their antiseptic, anti-infectious, and anti-viral properties. They create an uplifting quality and are regarded as non-toxic. Most alcohols in essential oils have a sweet, green, or sometimes woodsy smell and are light and pleasant.

PHENOLS – are very similar to alcohols with the exception that they normally have a more biting and medicinal smell. Phenols are analgesic, antiseptic, anti-infectious, antispasmodic, antiviral, bactericidal, digestive, diuretic, expectorant, sedative, and immune system stimulants. However, oils high in Phenols are considered the most irritating oils for the skin and mucous membranes and can cause dermatitis and sensitization. If phenols are present in high concentrations in an essential oil, that oil should be used in very low dilutions on the skin and only used for short periods. A few examples of these oils are clove, thyme, and basil.

OXIDES - oxides are most often used for their antiseptic, decongestant and expectorant properties. Oxides usually have fresh, sharp, and medicinal aromas. Some examples include: eucalyptus, rosemary, cajeput, and tea tree.

INGESTING ESSENTIAL OILS – THE BIG DEBATE

Can you take essential oils internally? That is the big question that has a lot of differing opinions. I hope that it is apparent that if one *were* to use essential oils this way that they must be pure, plant-base essential oils. The ingestion of artificial fragrance oil or essential oils that have been diluted with a chemical carrier could be fatal.

I admit that I do not promote the ingestion of essential oil in my business – mainly out of fear of public misuse. Many people are used to handling liquids in their kitchen such as vanilla extract, where they usually use an entire teaspoon in whatever they are concocting. Essential oils are vastly stronger than extracts. I would absolutely NEVER take one-eighth of a teaspoon of any essential oil – let alone and *entire* teaspoon!

I can tell you the way that I have personally used essential oils for internal use – in baking. Once, I made a chocolate cake and used only four drops of peppermint oil in the cake batter. I can tell you that small amount was sufficient for creating a chocolate-mint cake. When making lavender cookies, I use a single drop of lavender in the dough. Of course, with most lavender cookie recipes you see the addition of lavender buds, which I always use. But even with the dried flowers, using too much creates cookies that

51

taste like you are eating perfume. I have also used two drops of sweet orange essential oil in sugar cookie dough with good results and was definitely able to taste the orange. It is small amounts that create a subtle culinary difference in a recipe.

There are some oils that are used in meat dishes to replace dried herbs. Where you might usually sprinkle a little dried rosemary on top of chicken before baking and grilling it, using more than a single drop of rosemary this way can be overpowering and ruin the dish. One drop of rosemary diluted in olive oil or butter to glaze your chicken is plenty of rosemary flavor. Two drops tastes like you just took a bite out of a rosemary bush.

Aside from cooking, I have used essential oils internally when under the weather - but only on rare occasion. Whenever I get a simple toothache, I place a single drop of clove bud oil on my index finger then rub the gum next to the aching tooth. It usually gives instant relief but I can tell you that even that solitary drop makes your mouth feel numb (not for continuous daily use – twice a day, tops). During times of a sore throat, I've added a drop of peppermint oil to a small glass of water and gargled with it.

But, not all essential oils can be used this way. Some are extremely toxic and can cause vomiting, internal bleeding, and even death. A short list of the essential oils to always AVOID for internal use is: bitter almond, camphor, cassia, mugwort, pennyroyal, wintergreen, and wormwood. This is not a complete list. Once again, do a lot of reading and research from a variety of sources and when in doubt -just don't do it!

"THERAPEUTIC GRADE" ESSENTIAL OILS – WHAT DOES IT MEAN?

There has been no greater disservice to the field of aromatherapy and the use of essential oils than the term 'therapeutic grade'. No such grade exists. It is simply a marketing term – nothing else. It is a way for a company to advertise their essential oils as super-duper quality – better than the "other guy", a way to convince you that you'd better spend your money with them. They are better-stronger-faster, the Bionic Brand of essential oils. Not true.

There is no governing body that regulates or grades essential oils. Furthermore, there is no organization or defined set of standards that divide essential oils into specific grades. Once again, these are marketing phrases, used primarily by multi-level-marketing companies in their literature to encourage purchase of their essential oil products at a greatly inflated price - which, in turn, greatly inflates their profit margin. I am not going to mention any companies by name but a little research will show all you need to know about which companies sell essential oils in this manner.

I am sad to say, the people that sell them have fallen for the sales pitch most of the time. The last time I encountered one of these MLM representatives, I asked them, "Where did you learn about essential oils?" Their answer: the MLM company and ONLY the MLM company.   They had done no outside research on their own about essential oils and, prior to selling them for this company, had no previous experience or knowledge of essential oils. I asked if they had any books by other authors about essential oils. They did not.

The only thing they could continue repeating was that company's essential oils were superior because they are 'certified therapeutic grade' essential oils.

"Do you realize that in the United States that essential oils are not regulated or certified by anyone? There is no regulatory board or certification board," I said.

"That's not true," the sales rep insisted.   "Our company's essential oils are certified therapeutic grade!"

Just because a company goes out and registers the Trademark name 'certified therapeutic grade' doesn't make them certified or gives them the authority to create a non-existent grading system.   It may look fabulous on their brochures and sound great coming out of the mouths of their sales reps, but it isn't true. MLM companies must increase the price of a product greatly so they have room to "wholesale" to reps and "wholesale" again to the reps below them.   Why did I put the word *wholesale* in quotations? Because their "wholesale" price is above the normal retail price for essential oil companies that are not into multi-level marketing. It's a great way to get rich – convince people you are giving them a discount while you rake in the above-the-normal-retail-price big bucks. It's like marking up a $500 sofa to $1000 so you will look generous and bargain-worthy when a 30% OFF sign is placed on the middle cushion. Of course, with that discount, you just paid $700 for a $500 sofa!

Example: I want to start selling oranges. They cost me 50 cents each. To make a living, I am going to sell them to you for $1.00 each because that is the way business works. I have to sell them for more than I paid for them so I can pay my rent, utilities, food, etc.

Enter the MLM company wanting to sell oranges. They pay 50 cents for the orange just like I do. But, they want YOU and your friends below you to sell them, so they're going to give you 25% off the retail price of the orange. Then give you MORE if you sign up others to sell below you. But how will they profit? They are going to sell the oranges for $4.00 each instead of $1.00. How will they get away with this? Claim they are better than any orange in the world, superior in every way. They even go a step further and call their orange "certified tastiest and healthiest!" The people wanting to make 25% of $4.00 believe it (most of the time, because they *want* to believe it) and spread the fib to anyone who will listen.

Still, the MLM reps want to argue with you, telling you that they have visited and toured their company's lavender farm. Maybe so. But did they visit their patchouli farm? Their sandalwood forest? Their tropical ylang-ylang jungle? No. Because there is not enough land available for purchase in all parts of the world to supply an essential oil company with every plant they will need to make all of their oils. Some countries have farms that have been in the essential oil business for over one hundred years. They wholesale the oils to many companies, large and small.

Go out and ask farmers who produce plants for essential oil (and who are distilling their own) if they are sending off samples to the FDA and receiving a certificate saying their oil meets 'therapeutic grade' standards. You won't find a single one because this practice is simply not happening.

So, if I had to define it on a personal level without thinking about how the term has been overused - what does therapeutic grade mean to me? It means that the essential oil is pure with no chemical additives, dilutions or carrier oils. Pure oil is pure oil. A bottle of lavender that has ONLY lavender in it is suitable to use in an aromatherapy (keyword, *therapy*, as in *therapeutic*) treatment.

Does this mean that I am saying all essential oils are created equal? Certainly not. I wouldn't expect the oil from a potted lavender plant growing on the back porch of a house in Ohio to be the same quality as the lavender in the fields of France. Climate and growing conditions have a great impact on the quality of the plant and the essential oil obtained from it.

There are tests to determine if essential oils are pure. The two most common are Gas Chromatography testing and the Mass Spectrometry test. In Gas Chromatography testing, the process partitions the components of the essential oil and produces a reading (in the form of a chromatogram) which makes it possible to compare to known essential oil components. The essential oil slides through tubing (mixing with or sometimes forced through the tub by means of a gas compound) and upon evaporation, the trace of essential oil is measured. In other words, the essential oils are separated and vaporized without any decomposition happening. The process will tell if there are any unnatural substances present in the oil.

The Mass Spectrometry test converts the essential oil into ions so that they can be moved about and manipulated by external electric and magnetic fields. The ions are sorted and separated according to their mass and charge. The separated ions are then measured and displayed onto a chart showing the different components. However, some terpenes are impossible to identify using only this method. Oftentimes, the Mass Spectrometry test is performed right after the Gas Chromatography test. When these two methods are combined, the test will usually be referred to as a GC/MS test.

But, many suppliers use this testing method, not just the one's selling the priciest essential oils. And remember, these tests were not performed by anyone that passes out a certificate stamping the oils as 'therapeutic grade.' The tests are simply what they are – tests to show if an oil is pure.

Getting to know your supplier and doing a little research on your own is much better than just taking the word of a glossy, color brochure. With that said, don't believe everything you read on the internet! There are several articles out there written by reps and the misinformed who think they have all the answers and their lengthy articles *sound* very impressive and believable. One particular long article I found mentioned, *"The purity of an oil is also measured when considering it for therapeutic certification; the oil must be completely free of synthetic chemicals and heavy metals in order to receive therapeutic certification."* I repeat, there is NO certification process. Their article also mentions how essential oils fall into three categories: cosmetic grade, food grade, and therapeutic grade. No, No, and double No. There is no governing body, agency, or watch-group that grades essential oils. It is simply more marketing hype, empty words meant to sell a product. Of course, when I reached the end of the article, what do you think I found? Yes, the writer was a sales rep for one of the above-mentioned multi-level-marketing companies, and went on to say how their oils really were the best to be found! Uh huh, right.

IF there was such a thing as having your essential oils certified, then an essential oil company would not be permitted to trademark the terms 'certified therapeutic' or 'certified therapeutic grade'. When you Trademark a word or phrase, you are claiming those words for yourself, usually to brand your company. For example, there are many certified organic farms growing organic vegetables, all of which go under inspection to insure their farming methods will permit their certification. BUT, no single farmer can Trademark the words, 'certified organic'. If they were allowed to do this, no other farmer growing under natural conditions would be able to call their organic produce 'certified organic'. Since there is no certification process for essential oils, it has left room for companies to Trademark terms that make their brand appear superior to all others. If I have not said it enough times already, NO ONE in the United States certifies or grades essential oils.

While we are on this topic, allow me to say something else. Please pick a company/supplier that is passionate about essential oils and aromatherapy. We were recently set up at a fairgrounds market and, in the booth behind us, a husband and wife team were representing one of those MLM essential oil companies. But, the thing is, they hardly had any essential oils with them - just a few bottles for sniffing, along with some diet supplements. Instead, they were passing out brochures and had posters that said,

'BE A PART OF OUR TEAM'! To me, that is not someone who has dedicated themselves to aromatherapy and essential oil use/education. They were only interested in recruiting more people to sell under them so they could make more money. I mean, if you're going to sell essential oils, and talk all day about essential oils – could you please be bothered enough to bring a few bottles with you to sell? If you don't have any on hand and the only thing you want to do is "sign me up", that says a great deal to me about where your passion lies – with the money. It goes without saying, that my tongue was sore from biting it all day every time I heard the words 'certified therapeutic grade' slide out of their mouths.

QUESTIONABLE THERAPIES – THE USE OF UNDILUTED ESSENTIAL OILS ON THE SKIN

Some companies promote the use of undiluted essential oils as a therapy where they drop the oils onto the client's spine and massage the oils in. True aromatherapy associations try to distance themselves from these "therapies", even going as far as denying membership into their aromatherapy organization if the practitioner performs these alternative and unproven methods.

One obvious problem when it comes to these therapies is the fact that most states require a practitioner to be a licensed massage therapist if they are going to rub the body of a client. At the time of this writing, there are only five states in the United States that do not require a license in massage therapy — Kansas, Minnesota, Oklahoma, Vermont, and Wyoming. It does not matter if you have the client's permission or not. In states that require a massage license, no rubbing or massaging means exactly that — NO massaging or rubbing, period.

Massage therapy as defined by the Massage Therapy Licensing Program and the Texas Department of State Health Services --*The manipulation of soft tissue by hand or through a mechanical or electrical apparatus for the purpose of body massage. The term includes effleurage (stroking), petrissage (kneading), tapotement (percussion), compression, vibration, friction, nerve strokes, and Swedish gymnastics.*

The State of Tennessee describes massage therapy as*: Massage/bodywork/somatic -The manipulation of the soft tissues of the body with the intention of positively affecting the health and well-being of the client.*

Another concern I have when it comes to these therapies is the high amount of essential oils used. When you pour essential oils directly on the spine using oils that create "heat", they are actually causing skin irritation. Just because there is a heating effect happening doesn't necessarily mean it is a good thing. One essential oil that is commonly used in these therapy sessions is wintergreen. Wintergreen consists mainly of the chemical methyl salicylate. Methyl salicylate is believed to be readily absorbed through human skin and can result in dangerously high blood levels of salicylic acid. If swallowed, it is fatal and should never be used topically on a pregnant woman. Some who take arthritis medication are already receiving a small dose of this chemical component and rubbing it straight into the skin can create a dosage higher than expected.

It is more likely a concern for the practitioner who is performing these sessions as their hands are coming into constant contact with skin-irritating and/or toxic oils. Having your massage therapist include a few drops of wintergreen in a massage blend is one thing since most people do not treat themselves to a massage every day. However, what if you are the person performing massage or undiluted essential oil therapy using these oils? An aggressive practitioner might schedule several appointments a day, each time putting oils (such as wintergreen) into their own system by means of massaging it into their clients. Some will argue that their "therapeutic grade" oils are the exception and completely safe – because they have been taught and *told* this by the oil company. I could easily distill poison ivy essential oil and tell you that because I made it myself that it would not cause skin irritation – but that wouldn't make it true. I can tell you that in the past when I have met people that perform these types of therapies, I have always noticed what terrible shape their hands are in – usually red, irritated, and sometimes cracked.

The best advice I can possibly give about these

therapies is to read, read, and read. Do not simply read the literature distributed by the companies promoting it. What good would that do? Read articles, reviews (good and bad) from several sources and let your conscience be your guide.

CERTIFIED AROMATHERAPIST

I have taken two courses over the years. On passing the first level, I became a Certified Aromatherapist. A few years later I took the extended course, conducted case studies, and learned anatomy and physiology to help me become a Certified Clinical Aromatherapist. Now that I have said all this I must tell you, a certification is not the same thing as a license. There are currently no government agencies that license aromatherapists. When you receive a certificate, it means that you have studied and passed the exams for a predetermined set of curriculum on the subject of aromatherapy from a school that was approved by one of the Aromatherapy Associations. Therefore, I am certified by the school that trained me but the State or Federal government has no set standards/curriculum for the practice of aromatherapy.

However, there are professional, non-profit associations that have paved the way for true aromatherapy and set the standards for aromatherapy certification. Two such organizations are the National Association of Holistic Aromatherapy (NAHA), based in the United States, and the Canadian Federation of

Aromatherapy (CFA). Both have set specific core curriculum standards in the field of aromatherapy. For the school to be NAHA or CFA approved as a recommended or accredited school, it must meet agreed upon standards.

While neither is an official government agency, both were formed to insure that people who called themselves 'aromatherapists' are actually qualified since no official regulations exist. Many agree that when aromatherapy does become recognized, these agencies will have already set the professional standards for certification.

There is often confusion about the terminology used in the regulation and recognition of practitioners. Licensing and Registration is usually controlled by a government agency. Certification, on the other hand, may be controlled by either a government body or a private organization. In the United States and Canada, aromatherapy certification is controlled by private organizations – not the government.

THE ESSENTIAL OIL MEDICINE CABINET

There have been many times over the years that customers and clients have asked me, "If you could only choose five essential oils to use, which ones would they be?" The answer is the same whether using essential oils for the first time or trying to create an essential oil "medicine cabinet." The five oils would be: lavender, peppermint, eucalyptus, lemon, and tea tree.

LAVENDER for general relaxation and stress, to place on bug bites and burns, blisters, rashes, sunburns and many skin irritations. Lavender is the main soap and the main essential oil I use in the bath, primarily for its relaxing properties. It is also a good oil for a restful night's sleep. Simply place two or three drops on a bare pillow, put the pillowcase back on, and see how well the lavender helps with rest or insomnia. It also seems to work quite well when the cat gets a little too playful and gives me a good scratch. A drop rubbed into the scratch (after a good washing) prevents that "cat scratch itch" and seems to help it heal much faster.

PEPPERMINT is the best thing for a tension headache. Just placed two or three drops on a cotton ball, cradle in the palms of your hands, and breathe in deeply. A normal tension headache will ease off in about ten minutes. When used in bath products it can have a cooling effect (too much will be irritating, though). Peppermint is a good stimulating oil when you need to feel invigorated or on those mornings when you just can't seem to wake up. Mix a drop in a half-teaspoon of olive oil and rub on the stomach when you have stomach cramps or an irritable belly. Out of mouthwash? Add one or two drops in a glass of water and gargle with it. Rinse again with pure water after.

EUCALYPTUS is great for sinusitis and for when you have a cold or the flu. It is one of the ingredients in the well-known Vicks Vapor Rub. Whenever there is a cold in our household, we fill up the oil burner with mainly water and about six drops of eucalyptus oil, allowing the scent to fill the house. At bedtime, I place eucalyptus in the vaporizer beside the bed (make sure you have a vaporizer that will handle essential oil use). Eucalyptus is also good for muscular aches, tendinitis, and swelling.

LEMON is not only good for cheering you up and lifting your spirits, it makes for an excellent ingredient in natural cleaning products. Just remember that it is one of the phototoxic oils, so don't use before going out in the sun or in a tanning bed. Some people have reported that a single drop several times a week will make warts go away but I have no personal experience with this. A few drops of lemon oil in the dishwater really helps to cut grease and increase the cleansing power of the soap you are using. Feeling down? Blend a few drops of lemon with a few drops of lavender and smell the relaxing and cheerful aroma. A few drops in your shampoo also helps with oily hair.

TEA TREE is the king of the antifungal essential oils. It can be used to aid the healing of fingernail and toe funguses and has excellent reports in improving athlete's foot. When used in skincare products, it is wonderful for acne and troubled skin. While I have no proof of it, we have many customers who tell us they buy our tea tree soap because it helps maintain the color of their tattoos. The indigenous Bundjalung people of eastern Australia use "tea trees" as a traditional medicine by inhaling the oils from the crushed leaves to treat coughs and colds. They also use the leaves to create a poultice for wounds.

Of course, I could never limit myself to ONLY five essential oils. They each have their own expertise in the plant world. I can tell you that the five I mentioned above are readily available in my medicine cabinet at home. Whenever a customer comes into our store wanting to start their essential oil collection but they only want to start with a few – these are the ones I suggest.

USING ESSENTIAL OILS TO SCENT THE HOME

Almost everyone loves fragrance in the home. Some buy candles, others use potpourri, fragrance oils, or even plug-in air fresheners. Using essential oils to replace artificial fragrance in the home is not only a natural and more "green" alternative, but it can also trigger fewer allergies and irritations than their chemical counterparts do.

Home scents tend to change with the seasons - light florals in the spring, fresh and fruity smells in the summer months, followed by spices in autumn and winter. Real essential oils can achieve all of this and even help elevate the mood in the household with their aromatherapy benefits.

Spring scent choices include lavender, clary sage, orange, tangerine, bergamot, jasmine, geranium, petitgrain, lemon, chamomile, grapefruit, and lime. In the spring, most people want the fresh scent of flowers and plants in the house. Mixing citrus oils with florals makes a fresh and pretty smell. Combined, they are both relaxing and cheering.

Summer scent choices include lime, orange, tangerine, grapefruit, bergamot, palmarosa, lemongrass, lemon eucalyptus, citronella, juniper berry, peppermint, spearmint, and rosemary. You will notice that we have repeated the citrus oil. However, this time we are going to mix them with essential oils that come from grasses, green plants, and berries. In fact, if you include a little lemon eucalyptus and citronella into your blends you will find that it repels mosquitoes and ticks.

Autumn and winter scent choices include clove, cinnamon, frankincense, patchouli, sandalwood, cedarwood, cypress, palmarosa, chamomile, orange, tangerine, grapefruit, bergamot, and lemon. A blend that is heavy on the palmarosa and chamomile with the slightest touch of cinnamon added will create a natural version of apples-and-cinnamon. True, it won't smell just like the fragrance oil but it will certainly be in the same family and natural, to boot. Citrus oils blended with cinnamon and cloves create a warm smell reminiscent of the holiday season.

Please keep in mind that there a no hard and fast rules for creating scents throughout the seasons. It is all a matter of personal taste. The oils I chose above create scents similar to those found in stores during specific times of the year, scent profiles that remind you of the fresh days of spring, the warm and juicy fruits of summer, and the comforting spices of those cold months of autumn and winter.

One of the most often asked questions I receive in our store is, "what can I use to make my teenage son's room smell better?" It is true – most teenage boys have bedrooms that smell like locker rooms. When you want to mix a blend of essential oils good for odors, the mints and eucalyptus types are king. However, most people do not want to use straight eucalyptus or white camphor because they have a medicinal smell. Adding spearmint into the mix creates a fresh and vibrant blend that masks unpleasant odors. Peppermint is an alternative, but I have always found the sweetness of spearmint to work better as a room deodorizer. Keep in mind that mints are a stimulant, so it would be better to use them in the morning. This will allow the essential oils to do their job but not keep anyone up at night. Blending lavender into the mix would not be a bad option to counteract the stimulating effects. (See recipe section for an odor-spray.)

Oil burners are a great way to spread the aroma of essential oils throughout the house. When I refer to an oil burner, I mean the type with a small bowl for a top and a reservoir for holding a tea light candle underneath. I prefer the soapstone oil burners because more water can be added to them easily. With the glass-top oil burners, pouring more cool water into a hot glass dish will crack it almost every time. Many retailers will try to tell you to pour straight oil into the top, mainly because they want you to use it all up and come back to buy more. I never suggest this to my retail customers. Giving them proper instructions and money-saving tips has created life-long customers that trust me. So, fill the bowl with mainly water and about twelve to fifteen drops of essential oil, light the tea light candle underneath and within minutes the house fills with aromatherapy scents.

Several drops (about ten to fifteen) sprinkled on a coffee filter is perfect for placing over air vents in the house. Every time the air conditioning or heat turns on, it fills the room with natural scent.

A subtle method of scenting the home is by filling small bowls with Epsom salts or sea salt that you have premixed with essential oils. This method is popular for people who have trouble sleeping. Several customers tell me they use this method with essential oils of lavender and clary sage (sometimes chamomile) and keep the bowl on the nightstand beside the bed. I have also used this method when I had a cold or the flu – except the essential oils I used were eucalyptus, white camphor, lavender, basil, and ravensara. When it is a mild cold, I may only use eucalyptus.

There are several diffusers on the market. The one I have used the most is "Scentball" by the Earth Solutions company. I was so impressed with them that we began carrying them in our retail store. The Scentball is a plug-in diffuser with a small grill on top. Tightly woven pads are slid under the grid where they are heated, dispersing the essential oils that you had dropped onto the pad. The longest-lived Scentball I owned lasted nine years. However, I always unplugged the unit when it was not in use, which undoubtedly lengthened its life.

The description on the Earth Solutions website is as such:

ScentBall Aromatherapy Diffusers enable you to enjoy beautiful, natural fresh fragrances, safely and with minimal effort.

Before ScentBall Aromatherapy Diffusers were launched, the only known affordable electric room fresheners were made with artificial fragrances. The ScentBall was itself, once a bug repellent diffuser and is now a natural air freshener. To provide consumers the option of selecting their own natural essential oils, Earth Solutions expanded the consumer choice from chemical fragrance air fresheners to a naturally derived plant extract - plug in wall aromatherapy diffusers.

Add 10-20 drops of oil to the refill pad and insert it onto the warming element on one of your ScentBall Aromatherapy Diffusers and plug into any outlet. Aromatherapy scents will begin to diffuse within 5 minutes.

Add essential oils as often as desired. ScentBall Aromatherapy Diffusers pads are reusable and each diffuser includes 5 extra long pads, ideal for large spaces.

I know what you are thinking. No, this was not a paid testimonial by Earth Solutions – it just happens to be my favorite aromatherapy diffuser.

You can also use your essential oils to spruce up old potpourri that has lost its scent. Most commercial potpourri scent comes from artificial fragrance oils so invigorate that lifeless potpourri that has been gathering dust in your den. If you have to buy new, choose the least scented so that you can cover it up with your natural oils. Making your own potpourri is another option. A simple bowl of pinecones you have collected from the neighbor's yard (ask first) is the only thing you really need. Some craft stores sell unscented potpourri, although this is not available in all areas. I knew someone years ago, that kept a wooden bowl filled with twigs collected from the back yard, and he would drop essentials oils onto the pile each morning. When he tired of the scent, he let them dry thoroughly and burned them outside in his fire pit – instant homemade incense!

THE AROMATHERAPY BATH

Bath water is my personal favorite way of using essential oils. After all, I own a bath company so there is never a short supply of aromatherapy bath salts, essential oils soaps, or herbal tub teas around our house.

It makes me sad when a customer tells me that they do not own a bathtub, only a shower. To me, that says a great deal about our society today – that we cannot slow down long enough to enjoy the relaxation and therapy of a hot bath. There is only enough time for a quick trip through the shower for basic hygienic reasons. How unromantic and clinical. I have never seen a movie where the romantic lead spread rose petals on the floor of the shower because they didn't own a tub.

Hippocrates, known as the Father of Medicine, learned about the healing properties of aromatic baths from the ancient Egyptians. He developed teachings about using water as a form of treatment, which he called hydrotherapy. Medicinal bathing is also called thalassotherapy or hydrotherapy (water cure). The name thalassotherapy may come from the ancient Greek thalassa (small sea).

When adding essential oils straight to the bath water, only use between five and seven drops. The tub may look like a large amount of water that could easily handle more, but this small amount is really all you need. For example, more than eight drops of peppermint in the tub makes it feel like you are bathing in deep heating rub – and not in a good way. Start out small and work your way up to a comfortable ratio of essential oils to water. Essential oils will float on top of the water in droplets so spread the surface of the water around with your hand before stepping into the tub.

A simple and time-honored way of creating an aromatic bath is by using bath salts. You can create your own at home with sea salt, Epsom salt, or a combination of both. A very basic recipe is:

1 cup Epsom salt
8 drops essential oil of choice
Mix well and store in glass jar or cut the recipe in half for a single bath.
Add half-cup bath salt to running bath water

It is as simple as that. There are many salt choices. Sea salt is readily available in higher end grocery stores. Plain table salt is not a good choice for bath salt as it is drying to the skin.

ESSENTIAL OILS AND PETS

I must tell you that pet aromatherapy is not my area of expertise. I did want to bring up the subject, if for no other reason than to keep someone from accidentally poisoning a beloved family pet.

Essential oils can be used for dogs in a variety of ways, from bathing to calming the nerves, to flea and tick prevention. Always dilute essential oils for use on a dog at 20% the amount used on a human. (If your own blend calls for five drops of lavender, then the dog only gets one drop).

Never use essential oils on cats, ferrets, birds, or fish.

Felines have no means of processing essential oils; their livers cannot filter them out so the oils build up and become toxic. It is my understanding that the same applies to pets such as ferrets. Keep heavy usage of diffused essential oils to a minimum.

For birds and fish, even breathing in a consistent supply of essential oils can be deadly (fish, by way of the fumes settling on the water). Do not use your aromatherapy diffuser in the same room as your birds or your fish tank.

If you have a pet other than mentioned above, it does not mean that they can safely use essential oils. There are numerous and more detailed resources about pets and essential oils. If in doubt, consult your veterinarian.

RECIPES

While I never intended this book to be a recipe book of aromatherapy and essential oils, I do feel that you need a few blends and recipes to get you started on your path.   There are numerous books and resources where you can find more.   Another reason, I have to admit, is that my next book on making bath and body products will be heavy in the recipe department.   My main objective with this book is to cover the ins-and-outs of essential oils and aromatherapy.   When you get comfortable with blending essential oils, it will be time to start creating your own recipes.

BATH OIL

Bath oil seems to have gone out of fashion but it is a wonderful experience. You can use virtually any carrier oil you want but go easy and only use about a third of a teaspoon of the finished product in the tub – that is plenty to leave your skin feeling soft and smooth.   Too much can be oily and make the tub slippery.

For a relaxation bath oil, blend together:
2 ounces of liquid oil (olive, jojoba, etc)
12 drops lavender essential oil
3 drops geranium essential oil
2 drops clary sage essential oil

Store in a glass or plastic bottle with cap. If you have used carrier oils that go rancid quickly, store in the refrigerator to make it last longer.

MASSAGE OIL

Many massage oils can be used as bath oil. When blending massage oil you want to try to pick carrier oils that blend into the skin instead of leaving a greasy barrier on the surface. We are going to use a single base oil in this recipe and create different massage oils with the essential oils we choose.

BASE: 2 ounces of sweet almond oil
In the base of sweet almond, mix in the essential oil blends listed below based on the effect you want to achieve:

SORE MUSCLE BLEND: 5 drops peppermint, 3 drops ginger, 5 drops sweet marjoram, 3 drops cypress.

ROMANCE BLEND: 8 drops sandalwood, 3 drops ylang-ylang, 3 drops patchouli, 4 drops lavender.

STRESS BLEND: 7 drops lavender, 3 drops cedarwood atlas, 4 drops lemongrass, 3 drops geranium.

PERFUME

The art of perfumery is an exact science, down to the precise drop so there are a million different formulas you can create. I always use a base of pure-grain alcohol because it is the closest thing in composition to perfumer's alcohol. However, not every State sells pure-grain alcohol (brand name Everclear). So, an alternative to it is vodka. The difference is that vodka has a water content while pure-grain is nothing but alcohol. (and, no...rubbing alcohol will not work for perfume)

1 ounce alcohol base
20 drops sandalwood
5 drops jasmine (or rose)
6 drops citrus (lemon, orange, or tangerine)

Blend all ingredients in glass bottle, shake well, and allow to sit for several days. Best, when allowed to rest for two weeks or more. You can test right away but the scent will be different as it ages.

HEADACHE RELIEF

Headaches usually fall under two main categories – tension or migraine. This blend will help with a little of both. Peppermint is well known for relieving a tension headache, pink grapefruit oil is said to shrink swollen capillaries, lavender is for relaxation, and ginger is for the nausea associated with migraine headaches.

Place one drop of each oil (peppermint, pink grapefruit, lavender, and ginger) onto a cotton ball. Cradle the cotton ball in both hands and take long deep breaths to inhale the scent from the oils. After four or five deep breaths, set cotton ball aside and sniff again as needed.

MEDITATION ANOINTING OIL BLEND

Certain essential oils have been used for centuries in

both prayer and meditation. This blend helps to put you in that specific "zone". Anointing oils are usually applied using a drop of the mixture on the forehead (the third eye).

In one teaspoon carrier oil (your choice) mix:
2 drops sandalwood essential oil
1 drop frankincense essential oil
1 drop cedarwood essential oil
1 drop myrrh essential oil

Blend well and use as an anointing oil or can also be applied to the wrists as a pulse-point perfume.

CALM SLEEP BLEND
3 drops lavender essential oil
1 drop chamomile essential oil
1 drop clary sage essential oil

Drop each of the oils onto a cotton ball and rub the cotton ball across the surface of your pillow. With this blend, I always tell people to take the pillowcase off their pillow first, rub on the blend, allow to sit for a few minutes and then pull the pillowcase back on. This way, essential oils are not in direct contact with your eyes and face while you sleep. It should last for several days. If you do not want to place on pillow, simply drop oils onto cotton ball and breathe in deeply before going to bed.

ATHLETES FOOT RESCUE
Take a teaspoon of witch hazel and combine with:

2 drops tea tree essential oil
1 drop lavender essential oil
1 drop patchouli essential oil
Wash feet and dry thoroughly. Apply mixture
between the toes and top of nail beds with a cotton
ball or cotton swab. Apply up to twice a day.

ATHLETES FOOT SOAK

Mix together 1 cup Epsom salts with:
6 drops tea tree essential oil
3 drops lavender essential oil
1 drop patchouli essential oil
Blend well and use a handful of the salt mix in a
nightly foot soak of warm water.   Be sure to dry feet
thoroughly after soaking.

ODOR CONTROL SPRAY

To make a spray for odors, get an eight-ounce bottle
with a spray top or mister.   You will need:
8-ounce sprayer bottle
1-ounce vodka or pure grain alcohol
15 drops eucalyptus essential oil
10 drops spearmint essential oil
15 drops lavender essential oil
Purified or distilled water

Vodka has higher water content than pure grain
alcohol but both will work well for making a spray.
First, put the vodka in the bottle, then the essential
oils, cap and shake well.   Then top off with water and
your simple spray in ready.   The reason for the
alcohol content is that it helps to disperse the

essential oils. Since essential oils do not blend with water, you will still need to shake this each time before use.

NATURAL INSECT REPELLENT

A few years ago, the Center for Disease Control put out a press release stating that lemon eucalyptus essential oil was the best, natural alternative to DEET. Regular eucalyptus will not do. It is the high citral content in the lemon eucalyptus oil that does the trick. I have found many recipes that sing praises for lemongrass oil but it is a weaker choice when compared to lemon eucalyptus and citronella. However, when combined with them it makes for a much more pleasant smelling spray. We are going to use the same directions as the previous recipe (odor control) to make a spray.

8-ounce sprayer bottle
1-ounce vodka or pure grain alcohol
15 drops lemon eucalyptus essential oil
15 drops citronella essential oil
15 drops lemongrass essential oil

Combine all ingredients in bottle, top off with water and shake well before every use. Spray on legs, arms, back of neck to keep mosquitoes and ticks away. Can even be used to spray the shrubbery surrounding your patio.

CARPET POWDER

This is a basic carpet powder like the ones you find in

stores everywhere. The main difference is the use of real essential oils instead of the usual overpowering fragrance found in the big box store.

1 cup baking soda
12 drops lavender essential oil
6 drops bergamot essential oil
5 drops eucalyptus or spearmint essential oil (your preference)

Mix essential oils together and drop into the baking soda by sifting completely with your hands, breaking up the lumps that the oils create. When fully incorporated, sprinkle onto the carpet, allow to sit for five or ten minutes then vacuum up.

(add your own notes/recipe here)

ESSENTIAL OIL GUIDE

The information listed in this essential oil guide comes from a wide variety of sources and many years of research by means of: aromatherapy textbooks, essential oil encyclopedias, books on essential oils, and courses on aromatherapy.

I have tried to present the information on each of these fifty-five essential oils in an orderly, easy to understand manner. The spiritual use of each oil is not based on any particular religion or practice and is spread out over a wide variety of them.

It cannot be stressed enough that you should not use aromatherapy and essential oils as a replacement for traditional medicine. The information provided in this section is not a tool for you to diagnose, treat, or remedy illness or disease.   When in doubt, consult your physician.

ALLSPICE
Botanical Name: pimenta officinalis
Aromatic Profile: earthy, sweet and spicy with a similar scent to clove and cinnamon
Origin: Cuba, Jamaica, Mexico
Perfumery Note: middle
Extraction Method: steam distilled

About: Some stories say that Columbus brought allspice back to Europe, thinking it was pepper. Other reports claim that the English came up with the term "allspice", as they thought it was a blend of cinnamon, nutmeg, and clove. The allspice tree is in the evergreen family and can grow to a height of sixty feet. It is the berries (or fruit) of the allspice tree that the culinary spice and essential oil come from. The leaves of the tree are often used in cooking, the same way one would use a bay leaf. However, most of the time, they are used to enhance the flavor when meats are smoked.

USES -
Mind: aphrodisiac, balancing, nervous tension, exhaustion, sense enhancing, warming
Body: antiseptic, colds, cramps, muscular aches, rheumatism, sedative
Spirit: often used for luck, gambling, and personal power

Safety Warnings: May irritate mucous membranes, possible skin irritant if not thoroughly diluted.   Avoid during pregnancy.

AMYRIS
Botanical Name: amyris balsamifera
Aromatic Profile: woodsy, similar to sandalwood but less exotic and with a peppery undertone
Origin: Haiti, Asia
Perfumery Note: base
Extraction Method: steam distilled

About: While it bears no relation to sandalwood, Amyris is most often known as "poor man's sandalwood" or by the name "West Indian Sandalwood". It is an excellent ingredient for use in making natural perfumes. Often blended with real sandalwood to "stretch the budget" in perfumery.

USES -
Mind: balancing, restful and soothing to nerves, grounding, aphrodisiac
Body: muscle relaxant, soothing agent, slight sedative properties
Spirit: sensuality, romance, 4th chakra (heart), inner contemplation and meditation

Safety Warnings: Most sources list amyris as being non-toxic and non-irritating. However, it is a fairly "new" oil when it comes to aromatherapy so always perform a small patch test.

ANGELICA ROOT
Botanical Name: angelica officinalis
Aromatic Profile: woodsy, peppery, herbaceous
Origin: Belgium, France, Germany, Holland, Siberia
Perfumery Note: base
Extraction Method: steam distilled

About: Angelica is said to be a plant of divine origins, a perfume of the angels. It is said to have received its name because it bloomed around the feast day of the Archangel Michael. Angelica Root was believed to be a strong defense against all evil and witchcraft.

USES -

Mind: clear seeing – ability to see things for what they are, restful and soothing, strengthening, stress
Body: relieves nervous tension, asthma, bronchitis, carminative, colds, coughs, diuretic, expels mucous, estrogen-like, fainting, indigestion, immunity stimulant, influenza, menopause, migraines, postnatal depression, rheumatoid arthritis, toxin build-up, gout.
Spirit: Releases negativity. Said to ward off evil and bring luck in family matters.

Safety Warnings: Avoid during pregnancy. Avoid if diabetic. Phototoxic – stay out of sun during use.

ANISE

Botanical Name: pimpinella anisum
Aromatic Profile: sweet, licorice-like scent.
Origin: Mediterranean, Morocco, Spain
Perfumery Note: top
Extraction Method: steam distilled

About: Anise is an annual herbaceous plant that grows about three feet tall. It is a flowering plant that produces the sweet, licorice-tasting seeds called aniseed. It is not to be confused with star anise which is in the evergreen family. The seeds of the anise plant are used to make the liqueur anisette and are widely used to flavor foods, drinks, and candy.

USES -
Mind: cheering, energizing, euphoric, sense enhancing
Body: antibacterial, antispasmodic, bronchitis, colds,

flu, carminative, colic, coughs, cramps, deodorant, immunity stimulant, indigestion, lactation, hiccups.

Spirit: clairvoyance, divination, 6th chakra (third eye)

Safety Warnings: Avoid during pregnancy. Dilute well before use. Said to have narcotic-like properties and can slow circulation in large doses.

BASIL

Botanical Name: ocimum basilicum

Aromatic Profile: green, herbaceous scent with peppery undertones, slightly licorice-like in oil form

Origin: Europe, France, North America, Egypt

Perfumery Note: top

Extraction Method: steam distilled

About: A strong oil when used alone, it can be overpowering if not well-diluted or blended with another essential oil. Sweet Basil is the same plant that is used for culinary purposes and is most often associated with making pesto. Lovers of this dish will recognize the greenish-peppery scent of the essential oil.

USES -

Mind: exhaustion, mental fatigue, anxiety, encouragement, inspirational, cheering

Body: allergies, cold, coughs, bronchitis, withdrawals, PMS mood swings, circulatory stimulant, anti-bacterial, anti-viral, expectorant, gout, rheumatism, emphysema, whooping cough.

Spirit: money, prosperity, success in business.

Sometimes used for protection.

Safety Warnings: Avoid during pregnancy or if history of high blood pressure. Avoid if prone to seizures or a history of estrogen-dependent cancer.

BERGAMOT

Botanical Name: citrus bergamia
Aromatic Profile: an orange/lemon like scent with a dash of floral notes to it. A sophisticated citrus-like scent.
Origin: Italy, Morocco
Perfumery Note: top
Extraction Method: cold-pressed or steam distilled

About: Not only is bergamot good for a wide variety of skin irritations, it has been known to calm people with psychological disorders, including helping with depression and anxiety.

USES -

Mind: aggression, confidence, creativity, stress, cheering, withdrawals.
Body: boils and abscesses, chickenpox, mumps, cold sores, herpes, itching, oily skin, eczema, psoriasis.
Spirit: happiness, protection, success

Safety Warnings: Phototoxic, do not use before sunbathing or before a day in the sun. May irritate sensitive skin if not diluted properly.

CAJEPUT

Botanical Name: melaleuca cajeputi
Aromatic Profile: mainly camphorous but slightly fruit-like.
Origin: North America
Perfumery Note: middle
Extraction Method: steam distilled

About: In the tea tree family, cajeput is most often used during the cold and flu season. Also known to have pain killing properties and a single drop on a painful tooth can dull the pain until reaching a dentist. Can be blended well with a carrier oil and rubbed on the front of the neck to help with the pain of a store throat.

USES -
Mind: stimulating, energizing, focus
Body: colds, coughs, bronchitis, muscle aches, sinusitis, decongestant, temporary toothache pain reliever, sore throat.
Spirit: purification, self-awareness

Safety Warnings: Do not use during pregnancy. Avoid contact with mucous membranes. Possible skin irritation.

CAMPHOR, WHITE
Botanical Name: cinnamonum camphora
Aromatic Profile: strong and clean scent, similar smell to eucalyptus, cooling aroma
Origin: China, Japan, India
Perfumery Note: middle

Extraction Method: steam distilled

About: White camphor makes a good addition to massage blends to sooth sore muscles and arthritis. Can also be used as a decongestant whenever a cold or the flu comes around.

USES -

Mind: energizing, stimulating, nerves
Body: analgesic, anti-inflammatory, antiseptic, arthritis, bruises, burns, colds, coughs, decongestant, deodorant, disinfectant, gout, influenza, muscle relaxant,
Spirit: protection, psychic energy, 7th chakra (crown)

Safety Warnings: Do not take internally. Avoid if pregnant or epileptic. Not to be confused with the toxic oils of brown camphor, yellow camphor or borneo camphor. Do not use over long periods of time.

CARDAMOM
Botanical Name: elletaria cardamomum
Aromatic Profile: a sweet and spicy aroma, woodsy
Origin: Guatemala, India, Central America
Perfumery Note: middle
Extraction Method: steam distilled

About: Cardamom is a popular spice used all over the world. The essential oil has a pleasing scent that can give depth and a unique quality to essential oil blends. It is especially good when blended with citrus oils like orange and tangerine.

USES -
Mind: concentration, stimulating, depression, stress, fatigue
Body: appetite suppressant, circulatory stimulant, coughs, digestive, indigestion, infections, headaches, muscle relaxant, nausea, raises blood pressure,
Spirit: passion, love, and sex

Safety Warnings: Avoid if there is a history of high blood pressure.

CARROT SEED
Botanical Name: daucus carota
Aromatic Profile: strong, earth aroma; warm, sweet
Origin: Europe, England, France
Perfumery Note: middle
Extraction Method: steam distilled

About: Carrot seed oil is widely used in skincare formulas because of its skin repairing properties. Often found in wrinkle and anti-aging creams.   The scent alone is not particularly pleasing but blends well with other oils without dominating the other oils. Especially good for damaged and mature skin.

USES -
Mind: restoring, balancing, replenishes the thought process
Body: anti-inflammatory, calluses, chapped skin, corns, dandruff, dermatitis, dilates blood vessels, dry

skin, eczema, fragile hair, gout, hair loss, hangovers, normalizes skin, rashes, rosacea, skin conditioner, skin toner, soothing agent, wrinkles
Spirit: healing energy, unblocking negativity and old habits

Safety Warnings: Do not use during pregnancy.

CEDARWOOD ATLAS
Botanical Name: cedrus atlantica
Aromatic Profile: rich, sweet, woody
Origin: Algeria, Morocco, Himalayas
Perfumery Note: base
Extraction Method: steam distilled

About: The Atlas Cedar trees are tall and can live for centuries. In ancient times it was used to construct coffins and was also used by the Egyptians as an ingredient in the embalming process. A popular oil that predates Biblical times and was one of the first oils to be extracted. Cedarwood works well in masculine blends because of its woodsy aroma and is often used in perfumery. While it has positive effects on the skin, it should be used in low doses –
preferably blended with other essential oils. Can bring a rich quality to an essential oil blend.

USES -
Mind: positive state of mind, stabilizes the emotions, brings harmony, focus, stress
Body: acne, air purifier, antiseptic, antispasmodic, arthritis, bronchitis, cellulite, constipation, coughs,

dandruff, eczema, hair loss, immunity stimulant, insect repellent, oily skin, osteoarthritis, psoriasis, rheumatism

Spirit: meditation, psychic energy, spirituality, unhexing, associated with 4th chakra (heart) but also works well with the 7th chakra (crown)

Safety Warnings: Do not use during pregnancy. May irritate sensitive skin so dilute well.

CHAMOMILE, GERMAN

Botanical Name: matricaria chamomilla
Aromatic Profile: sweet, fruity, slightly reminiscent of apples
Origin: Hungary, Eastern Europe
Perfumery Note: middle
Extraction Method: steam distilled

About: Also known as blue chamomile due to the color of the essential oil. Good for the treatment of allergies such as eczema, urticaria and all dry, flaky and itchy condition. Also useful for treating sunburn and blemished skin, and in many cases has helped with dermatitis and psoriasis. If used in a blend solely for the purpose of smell, keep in mind that chamomile can quickly take over an entire blend with its scent. Start with a few drops and build from there until the desired scent is reached.

USES -
Mind: restful and soothing, relaxing, nerves
Body: acne, analgesic, antibacterial, antidepressant,

anti-inflammatory, antiseptic, antispasmodic, asthma, black eyes, blisters, boils, bruises, burns, chapped lips, chapped skin, disinfectant, diuretic, dry skin, earaches, eczema, fainting, fibrositis, hay fever, headaches, heatstroke, hiccups, influenza, insect bites, laryngitis, migraines, nausea, neuralgia, normal skin, oily skin, psoriasis, rashes, rheumatism, rheumatoid arthritis, rosacea, sensitive skin, shock, sprains, sunburns, toothaches, uticaria, wounds, wrinkles, skin inflammations

Spirit: peaceful thoughts, sleep and dreams, 5th chakra (throat)

Safety Warnings: Do not use during first trimester of pregnancy. Avoid if allergic to ragweed and pollen.

CHAMOMILE, ROMAN

Botanical Name: anthemis nobilis
Aromatic Profile: sweet and fruity with a hint of a woody and herbaceous scent
Origin: France, Belgium, Britain, North America
Perfumery Note: middle
Extraction Method: steam distilled

About: Roman chamomile is often used as a nerve sedative and is effective when used in blends for stress and anxiety. Has been used throughout history as a hot compress for skin abscesses and boils, as well as for soothing skin rashes. Can be used as a cold compress for sprains and pulled tendons.

USES -

Mind: restful and soothing, relaxing, creativity,

Body: all-purpose anti-inflammatory, acne, analgesic, antibacterial, antidepressant, antiseptic, antispasmodic, black eyes, blisters, boils, bruises, burns, bursitis, chapped lips, chapped skin, chilblains, cold sores, disinfectant, diuretic, dry skin, eczema, endometriosis, fainting, headaches, hiccups, insect bites, insomnia, laryngitis, migraines, nausea, neuralgia, nervine, psoriasis, rashes, rheumatism, rheumatoid arthritis, shock, sprains, stress, sunburns, toothaches, uticaria

Spirit: the same as German chamomile, it is used for peaceful thoughts, sleep and dreams

Safety Warnings: Do not use during first trimester of pregnancy. Avoid if allergic to ragweed and pollen.

CINNAMON LEAF

Botanical Name: cinnamomum zeylancium
Aromatic Profile: spicy, warm, the oil smells clove-like
Origin: Indonesia, Sri Lanka, Madagascar
Perfumery Note: middle
Extraction Method: steam distilled

About: Most often, the cooking spice called cinnamon that is found in the grocery store is not cinnamon at all but a close relation called cassia. This is why most people are surprised that the oil smells more like clove than the cinnamon smell they are accustomed to. Cinnamon leaf is easily found but cinnamon bark oil is available, yet, expensive.

Cinnamon essential oil can irritate the skin and should be heavily diluted and is usually not used in products that remain on the skin, such as lotion.

USES -

Mind: aphrodisiac, energizing, invigorating, refreshing, stimulating

Body: antibacterial, antibiotic, antifungal, antiseptic, antispasmodic, antiviral, bronchitis, colds, influenza, lice, muscular aches, rheumatism, scabies, stress, warts, whooping cough

Spirit: money, business success, prosperity, protection, 1st chakra (root)

Safety Warnings: Avoid during pregnancy. Not for use on young children. Possible skin irritant. Mucous membrane irritant. Avoid if a history of high blood pressure or if using blood thinning medication.

CITRONELLA

Botanical Name: cymbopogon nardus
Aromatic Profile: grassy, citrus-like, fresh, lemon-like, and sweet
Origin: China, Indonesia, South America
Perfumery Note: top
Extraction Method: steam distilled

About: Citronella is best known for its insect repelling properties. This property has been backed by studies and is especially good for warding off mosquitoes. Some say it is helpful in soothing barking dogs and is often found in natural dog shampoos.

USES -
Mind: fatigue, stimulating, refreshing,
Body: antiseptic, arthritis, colds, deodorant, diuretic, influenza, insect repellent, moth repellent, oily skin, perspiration, rheumatism, head and body lice
Spirit: cleansing, purification, unhexing, washing away negative energy

Safety Warnings: Avoid during pregnancy

CLARY SAGE
Botanical Name: salvia sclarea
Aromatic Profile: herbaceous, woodsy, slightly fruit-like
Origin: Russia, France, North America
Perfumery Note: middle
Extraction Method: steam distilled

About: Clary sage is a biennial plant, which means it lives for only two years. It has been used throughout the centuries as a medicinal plant and is also found in perfumes and some wines and liqueurs. Clary sage is said to mimic the female hormone which is why it is avoided by those who have had breast or ovarian cysts. Said to be the best oil for writers to increase their creativity and productivity.

USES -
Mind: anxiety, aphrodisiac, balancing, restful and soothing, fatigue, fear, nervous tension, stress, visualizing
Body: acne, anticonvulsive, antidepressant, anti-

inflammatory, antiseptic, antispasmodic, asthma, astringent, boils, bronchitis, cramps, dandruff, deodorant, dry skin, estrogen-like, female infertility, hot flashes, menopause, migraines, muscle relaxant, muscular aches, PMS symptoms, sedative, varicose veins, wrinkles

Spirit: vivid dreaming, 6th chakra (third eye)

Safety Warnings: Avoid during pregnancy, history of low blood pressure or estrogen-dependent cancer. Avoid consumption of alcohol during use. Avoid if there is a history of breast or ovarian cysts

CLOVE BUD

Botanical Name: eugenia caryophyllata
Aromatic Profile: spicy, sweet, hot
Origin: Indonesia, India, Pakistan
Perfumery Note: base
Extraction Method: steam distilled

About: Clove oil has been used in dentistry for years to dull the pain of a toothache. A single drop of clove essential oil on an aching tooth temporarily relieves the pain. Clove buds are one of the most used spices all over the world but are most often used in Middle Eastern cooking. Clove essential oil is useful as an ant repellent.

USES -
Mind: memory loss, concentration, sharpens the senses, stimulates the mind
Body: analgesic, antibacterial, antibiotic, antiseptic,

antispasmodic, antiviral, arthritis, asthma, bronchitis, colds, flatulence, frostbite, heartburns, insect repellent, moth repellent, muscle relaxant, nausea, neuralgia, osteoporosis, raises blood pressure, rheumatism, sprains, toothaches
Spirit: divination, psychic awareness, courage, balances chakras

Safety Warnings: Avoid during pregnancy. Avoid if a history of high blood pressure. Dilute well, may be skin irritant.

CORIANDER
Botanical Name: coriandrum sativum
Aromatic Profile: spicy and sweet with a faint scent of balsam
Origin: Southern Europe, Greece, India, North America
Perfumery Note: middle
Extraction Method: steam distilled

About: The fruit, or coriander seeds are from the cilantro plant. These two components of one plant have completely different tastes – the seeds being warm and nutty and the cilantro leaves are green and peppery. Coriander has been cultivated for centuries – grown purposely in ancient Greece and is found wild and plentiful all over Southern Europe. It appeared in North America when early colonists brought it over around 1670.

USES -

Mind: aphrodisiac, clarifying, creativity, energizing, exhaustion, fatigue, refreshing, stimulating, stress, warming

Body: anti-inflammatory, anti-spasmodic, arthritis, circulatory stimulant, colds, colic, cramps, gout, indigestion, muscle relaxant and pains, rheumatism

Spirit: healing energy

Safety Warnings: Avoid during pregnancy. Avoid if a history of high blood pressure or breast cancer.

CYPRESS

Botanical Name: cupressus sempervirens

Aromatic Profile: evergreen, herbaceous, fresh, clean

Origin: Mediterranean, Europe

Perfumery Note: middle

Extraction Method: steam distilled

About: Cypress is a tall evergreen tree that is native to the Mediterranean but it also popular in formal English gardens and around temples in Asia. The leaves have a scale-like appearance. Cypress is a popular essential oil to use in massage therapy blends because of its effectiveness on muscle aches and cramps.

USES -

Mind: aggression, balancing, irritability, nervous tension, refreshing, restlessness

Body: amenorrhea, antibacterial, anti-infectious, antiseptic, antispasmodic, antiviral, arthritis, asthma, astringent, broken capillaries, bruises, bronchitis, cellulite, circulatory stimulant, coughs, cuts, dandruff, deodorant, heavy menstruation, hemorrhoids, hot flashes, menopause, muscular aches, muscular cramps, noise pollution, normal skin, oily hair, oily skin, raises blood pressure, rheumatism, sinusitis, tennis elbow, varicose veins, excessive perspiration, loss of liquid in the body

Spirit: protection, healing, blessing, purification

Safety Warnings: Avoid during pregnancy. Avoid if a history of high or low blood pressure.

EUCALYPTUS

Botanical Name: eucalyptus globulus
Aromatic Profile: fresh, clean, camphorous
Origin: Spain, Australia, Tasmania
Perfumery Note: top
Extraction Method: steam distilled

About: Eucalyptus is probably the most popular essential oil when it comes to cold and flu season. While there are many other wonderful oils for these ailments, eucalyptus is the oil everyone has heard of and, therefore, the one they reach for. Great for opening up the sinuses and working as a decongestant.

USES -

Mind: balancing, cooling, refreshing, revitalizing
Body: analgesic, antibacterial, antibiotic, antifungal, anti-inflammatory, antiseptic, antispasmodic, antiviral,

bedbugs, bronchitis, chapped lips, circulation, colds, coughs, cystitis, dandruff, decongestant, deodorant, diarrhea, disinfectant, diuretic, drug withdrawal, flatulence, hay fever, heartburns, heatstroke, insect bites, jet lag, lice, lower abdominal pain, muscular aches, muscular dystrophy, muscular fatigue, neuralgia, normal hair, osteoarthritis, pneumonia, rheumatoid arthritis, sinusitis, stomachaches, sunburns, swelling, tendinitis, tennis elbow, urticaria, windburns

Spirit: psychic energy, health, protection

Safety Warnings: Avoid if using homeopathic remedies or if there is a history of epilepsy

EUCALYPTUS, LEMON – LEMON EUCALYPTUS

Botanical Name: eucalyptus citriodora
Aromatic Profile: lemony, fruity, sweet, woody
Origin: Australia, Tasmania
Perfumery Note: middle
Extraction Method: steam distilled

About: Lemon eucalyptus is probably the best insect repellent of all the essential oils, even more effective than citronella. The scent if very similar to citronella. According to the CDC, lemon eucalyptus oil is a safe and natural alternative to DEET. Good for keeping away mosquitoes and ticks and works well when added to dog shampoos. Lemon Eucalyptus has almost all of the same benefits of eucalyptus oil, although eucalyptus globulus is better for sore muscles.

USES -

Mind: balancing, cooling, refreshing, revitalizing

Body: analgesic, antibacterial, antibiotic, antifungal, anti-inflammatory, antiseptic, antispasmodic, antiviral, bedbugs, bronchitis, circulation, colds, coughs, cystitis, dandruff, decongestant, deodorant, diarrhea, disinfectant, diuretic, drug withdrawal, flatulence, hay fever, heartburns, heatstroke, insect bites, jet lag, lice, muscular aches, muscular dystrophy, muscular fatigue, neuralgia, osteoarthritis, pneumonia, rheumatoid arthritis, sinusitis, stomachaches, sunburns, swelling, windburns

Spirit: healing, house blessing, protection

Safety Warnings: Avoid if using homeopathic remedies or if there is a history of epilepsy

FRANKINCENSE

Botanical Name: boswellia carterii

Aromatic Profile: rich, woody, hint of spicy, fruity

Origin: Africa, Ethiopia, India

Perfumery Note: base

Extraction Method: steam distilled

About: Frankincense is also known as olibanum. Similar to the way trees are tapped for the making of maple syrup, the bark of the Boswellia tree is slashed and the resin is allowed to drip out and harden. This is what is known as Frankincense tears. The essential oil is richer, deeper and sweeter in smell than the resin it comes from and has been used in perfumery and to make incense. It is mentioned in the Hebrew Bible as one of the consecrated incenses. It is still used today for spiritual purposes.

USES -

Mind: anxiety, restful and soothing, clarifying, clearing, exhaustion, focusing, grounding, stress
Body: abrasions, antidepressant, antiseptic, asthma, astringent, cirrhosis of liver, diarrhea, diuretic, normal skin, oily skin, rheumatoid arthritis, scars, sedative, skin conditioner, varicose veins, wrinkles
Spirit: blessing, consecration, meditation, purification, 3rd chakra (solar plexus), spirituality

Safety Warnings: Avoid during pregnancy

GALBANUM

Botanical Name: ferula galbaniflua
Aromatic Profile: fresh, clean, green, earthy, woody
Origin: Middle East, Lebanon
Perfumery Note: top
Extraction Method: steam distilled

About: Like Frankincense, Galbanum is mentioned in the Hebrew Bible as one of the consecrated incenses. It is the gum resin of the Persian plant ferula gummosa, a large perennial herb that can grow as tall as six feet and is related to parsley. Galbanum is used in perfumery to give a fresh "green" scent to blends. It is highly used in anti-aging products to tone the skin and smooth wrinkles.

USES -
Mind: energizing, awakens the mind, stimulates the thought process
Body: abscesses, acne, anti-inflammatory, anti-spasmodic, antiviral, bronchitis, muscle relaxant, scars, skin conditioner, swelling, toning, wounds, wrinkles
Spirit: forgiveness, repentance

Safety Warnings: Avoid during pregnancy as this oil stimulates menstruation

GERANIUM
Botanical Name: pelargonium graveolens
Aromatic Profile: floral, sweet, and fruity
Origin: Egypt, South Africa
Perfumery Note: middle
Extraction Method: steam distilled

About: The essential oil is highly used in the perfume industry because it wears many masks when it comes to smell – rose-like, fruity, and slightly citrusy. The flowers and the leaves of the plant are sometimes used for culinary purposes such as jellies and jams, cakes, and ice cream. Unfortunately, geranium is sometimes used to adulterate rose oil. In aromatherapy, it is very helpful during times of grief.

USES -
Mind: anxiety, creativity, grief, nervous tension,

relaxing, self-hypnosis, soothing, stress

Body: acne, Alzheimer's disease, analgesic, antibacterial, antidepressant, antifungal, antiseptic, antispasmodic, antiviral, asthma, astringent, black eyes, blisters, blood disorders, broken capillaries, bruises, cellulite, chapped lips, chapped skin, circulatory stimulant, cold sores, constipation, cramps, diabetes, diarrhea, dry hair, dull skin, endometriosis, female infertility, hair loss, hay fever, herpes, hot flashes, immunity stimulant, laryngitis, lice, lower abdominal pain, menopause, muscular dystrophy, normal hair, normal skin, oily skin, osteoporosis, Parkinson's disease, PMS symptoms, rheumatoid arthritis, sedative, shock, varicose veins

Spirit: happiness, protection, used during times of grief to calm and cheer

Safety Warnings: Avoid if a history of hypoglycemia or estrogen-dependent cancer

GINGER

Botanical Name: zingiber officinale
Aromatic Profile: spicy, woodsy, smoky
Origin: South Africa, East Asia, Caribbean
Perfumery Note: middle/base
Extraction Method: steam distilled

About: Ginger has been used for centuries as a spice and a medicine. It is the rhizome of the plant and related to cardamom. Above the ground, the plant has reed-like stems that grow to a height of around 3 to 4 feet. It is used in a culinary capacity to make ginger ale and gingerbread. Ginger tea helps reduce nausea and motion sickness, as does smelling the essential oil of ginger.

USES -
Mind: energizing, memory boosting, grounding, stimulating
Body: antiseptic, antispasmodic, appetite stimulant, arthritis, bronchitis, bursitis, carminative, chills, circulation, colds, coughs, diarrhea, exhaustion, flatulence, hangovers, indigestion, laryngitis, motion sickness, muscular aches, nausea, normalizes blood pressure, osteoarthritis, osteoporosis, parasiticide, pneumonia, rheumatoid arthritis, sea sickness, sprains, tendinitis, tennis elbow, tonsillitis, travel sickness, vomiting
Spirit: attraction, lust, sex, prosperity, energy

Safety Warnings: Slightly phototoxic

GRAPEFRUIT
Botanical Name: citrus paradisi
Aromatic Profile: sweet, fruity, citrusy, bright
Origin: North America, Barbados
Perfumery Note: top
Extraction Method: cold pressed/expressed

About: When people think about eating grapefruit, they think of the bitter, tart taste it has. Essential oil of grapefruit is much sweeter and blends well with so many other essential oils. This citrus tree is a hybrid that was first bred in Barbados in the 18th century and is a descendent of the sweet orange and the pomelo fruit. Grapefruit is said to shrink capillaries, therefore it is put to good use when included in blends for migraine headaches.

USES -
Mind: concentration, creativity, energizing, inspiring, invigorating, refreshing, reviving, stimulating, stress, inspirational
Body: antibacterial, antidepressant, astringent, cellulite, diuretic, drug withdrawal, exhaustion, hangovers, jet lag, migraines, muscular aches, muscular fatigue, PMS symptoms, toxin buildup, water retention
Spirit: new beginnings, purification

Safety Warnings: Phototoxic, do not use before spending a day in the sun

HELICHRYSUM
Botanical Name: helichrysum italicum
Aromatic Profile: herbaceous, earthy, fresh, green-like scent
Origin: Africa, Madagascar, Australia, New Zealand
Perfumery Note: base
Extraction Method: steam distilled

About: Helichrysum is thought to be the most healing of all the essential oils. Many are surprised to find out that it is in the sunflower family. It is also known as Everlasting or Immortelle oil and has a very long shelf life. Rather expensive oil but an important addition to the aromatherapy medicine cabinet.

USES -
Mind: positive thoughts, relaxing, cheering, unresolved emotional issues
Body: anti-inflammatory, anticoagulant, antispasmodic, abscesses, acne, asthma, boils, burns, cuts, dermatitis, headaches, roseacea, bruising, scarring, back pain, eczema, rheumatoid arthritis, bursitis, circles under eyes, chigger bites, irritated skin, irritated bowels
Spirit: banish negativity

Safety Warnings: No special precautions noted. Always do a small patch test on the skin with any essential oil to see how it interacts with your body.

JASMINE ABSOLUTE
Botanical Name: jasminum grandiflorum
Aromatic Profile: floral, sweet, exotic, rich, strong
Origin: Asia, India, Africa
Perfumery Note: middle
Extraction Method: solvent extracted

About: Jasmine is a plant in the olive family that is well-known for its highly fragrant blossoms. However, the jasmine petals are too delicate to withstand the steam distillation process. In the past, jasmine was obtained through enfleurage, a process in which animal fats are smeared onto glass along with plants (in this case, jasmine petals) to scent the fat. Today, jasmine is usually solvent extracted. This is why jasmine oil is classified as an absolute instead of an essential oil. The oil is extremely strong – a few drops goes a very long way.

USES -

Mind: aphrodisiac, anxiety, hypnotic, nerve restful and soothing, relaxing

Body: antidepressant, anti-inflammatory, antiseptic, antispasmodic, coughs, cramping, depression, dry skin, emollient, labor pains, lethargy, menopause, subtle analgesic, normal skin, oily skin, PMS symptoms, sedative, skin conditioner

Spirit: love, sex, attraction, opening psychic ability, shamanic journeying

Safety Warnings: Avoid overuse during pregnancy. Narcotic-like properties so use in small amounts

JUNIPER BERRY

Botanical Name: juniperus communis
Aromatic Profile: woodsy, earthy, fruity, dry
Origin: Europe, Italy, North America
Perfumery Note: middle
Extraction Method: steam distilled

About: Juniper berries are not actual berries, but rather the female seed cone of the juniper plant. In the culinary world, juniper is used to flavor the liquor known as gin and sometimes as a spice. Juniper has been used since ancient times and is even mentioned in the Bible. Juniper berries have also been found in Egyptian tombs, despite the fact that it was not found in that region. It has been used medicinally all over the globe, including the ancient Greeks and the Native Americans.

USES -

Mind: anxiety, clearing, energizing, exhaustion, memory, refreshing, stress

Body: antifungal, anti-infectious, antiseptic, antispasmodic, arthritis, astringent, bursitis, cellulite, circulatory stimulant, colds, deodorant, detoxifying, disinfectant, diuretic, ear infection, gout, hemorrhoids, influenza, jet lag, muscular aches, nervine, normal skin, oily skin, raises blood pressure, rheumatism, sinusitis, swelling, toning, toxic buildup, varicose veins, water retention

Spirit: purification, exorcism, purging negative thoughts, spirit guides

Safety Warnings: Avoid during pregnancy or a history of high blood pressure. Should be avoided by those with kidney disease.

LAVENDER

Botanical Name: lavandula officinalis
Aromatic Profile: floral, fresh, clean, herbaceous, slightly camphorus
Origin: France, Spain
Perfumery Note: middle
Extraction Method: steam distilled

About: Lavender is probably the most popular and well-known essential oil. It is most often used for relaxation and sleep but is wonderful on burns, bug bites, and stings. Besides its many aromatherapeutic uses, it is used as an ingredient in upscale cooking and can be found in: cakes, breads, cookies, ice cream, and even to flavor sugar and honey. In the beauty industry, lavender is commonly used in soaps, lotions, salves, and creams.

USES -

Mind: aggression, anxiety, balancing, restful and soothing, exhaustion, fatigue, hysteria, nervous tension, relaxing, soothing, stress

Body: abrasions, abscesses, acne, animal bites, antibacterial, antibiotic, antidepressant, antifungal, anti-inflammatory, antiseptic, antispasmodic, antiviral, blisters, boils, bruises, burns, chapped skin, chicken pox, colds, convalescence, coughs, cuts, dandruff, dermatitis, detoxifying, diaper rash, diarrhea, disinfectant, endometriosis, hay fever, headaches, heartburns, hiccups, immunity stimulant, influenza, insect bites, insect repellent, insomnia, itching, labor pains, migraines, muscular aches, neuralgia, normalizes skin, rashes, scabies, sedative, shock, sinusitis, sprains, sunburns, swelling, tendinitis, tonic, toothaches, ulcers, urticaria, windburn, wounds

Spirit: love, happiness, peace, 6th chakra (third eye), and helps to balance all chakras

Safety Warnings: Avoid during first trimester of pregnancy

LEMON

Botanical Name: citrus limonum
Aromatic Profile: fruity, citrus, light, tart
Origin: Asia, South America, North America
Perfumery Note: top
Extraction Method: steam distilled from peel / cold-pressed

About: Genetic studies shows that the lemon is a hybrid of the sour orange and the citron, and was first found in Southern India and China. Grown mainly for its culinary use, it is a main ingredient in the drink industry.

USES -
Mind: anxiety, balancing, restful and soothing, cheering, refreshing, relaxing, stimulates the mind, stress, inspirational
Body: abscesses, acne, antibacterial, antifungal, anti-infectious, antiseptic, antispasmodic, antiviral, arthritis, asthma, astringent, athlete's foot, blisters, boils, circulatory stimulant, cold sores, constipation, corns, coughs, detoxifying, diarrhea, digestive, disinfectant, diuretic, gallstones, gout, headaches, hiccups, hot flashes, mumps, muscular dystrophy, normal hair, normal skin, normalizes blood pressure, oily hair, oily skin, rheumatoid arthritis, sedative, shock, sore throat, tendinitis, thrush, toning, varicose veins, warts
Spirit: 3rd chakra (solar plexis), balances emotions, purification, health

Safety Warnings: Phototoxic – do not use before

going out in the sun, may irritate sensitive skin

LEMONGRASS

Botanical Name: cymbopogon citratus
Aromatic Profile: lemony, earthy, fresh, green
Origin: India, Asia, Brazil
Perfumery Note: top
Extraction Method: steam distilled

About: Lemongrass is a tall, perennial grass and is widely used in Asian cuisine. It is used a variety of ways: fresh, dried, chopped, powdered and is well-known as the main ingredient in a popular Thai soup. As far as its herbal properties, lemongrass is a natural deodorant and insect repellent. When used in essential oil blends, lemongrass can quickly take over the blend so it should be used in small quantities if the scent of the other oils will be allowed to come through.

USES -

Mind: cleansing, concentration, exhaustion, invigorating, irritability, mental fatigue, stress
Body: analgesic, anti-inflammatory, antidepressant, antifungal, antiseptic, arthritis, astringent, athlete's foot, bruises, cellulite, circulatory stimulant, excessive perspiration, deodorant, indigestion, insect repellent, jet lag, moth repellent, muscular aches, oily hair, oily skin, raises blood pressure, sedative, scabies, sprains
Spirit: psychic ability, spirituality

Safety Warnings: Avoid during pregnancy or a

history of high blood pressure. Somewhat phototoxic. Avoid in cases of glaucoma.

LIME

Botanical Name: citrus aurantifolia
Aromatic Profile: fruity, tangy, zesty, fresh, green
Origin: Mexico, Caribbean, North America
Perfumery Note: top
Extraction Method: steam distilled from peel, cold-pressed / expressed

About: Lime essential oil can bring a cheerful, bright scent to an ordinary essential oil blend. Unlike the other citruses like orange, tangerine, lemon, and grapefruit, it imparts a sweet and tangy quality that makes the mouth water. Lime can be extremely phototoxic and cause blistering if it is used before going out in the sun. Besides being a culinary item, it is known for adding a dry and fruity quality to perfume.

USES -
Mind: anxiety, cheering, concentration, energizing, exhaustion, refreshing, stimulating
Body: antibacterial, antibiotic, antidepressant, antiseptic, asthma, astringent, colds, dandruff, flu, headaches, normal skin, oily skin, rheumatism, varicose veins
Spirit: protection, purification, 4th chakra (heart), cleanses the aura

Safety Warnings: Phototoxic – do not use before

going out in the sun. May irritate sensitive skin.

LITSEA

Botanical Name: litsea cubeba
Aromatic Profile: rich, lemony, earthy, sharp, sweet
Origin: China, Malaysia
Perfumery Note: top/middle
Extraction Method: steam distilled

About: Litsea is also known as May Chang and the plant is a member of the laurel family. While it is very lemon-like, in the perfumery world it is sometimes considered a middle note because of its staying power. Litsea has many of the same natural, chemical components of lemon verbena which is why it smells very similar but is much more affordable.

USES -

Mind: restful and soothing, cheering, inspirational, mood balancing
Body: acne, antifungal, allergies, antibacterial, asthma, bronchitis, deodorant, eczema, sedative
Spirit: centers the emotions, calm dreams

Safety Warnings: Avoid if a history of glaucoma. Should not be used on children under 10 years of age. May irritate sensitive skin. Not for use with damaged skin.

MANDARIN

Botanical Name: citrus reticulata
Aromatic Profile: sweet, citrusy, fruit, bright

Origin: Brazil, China, Italy, Spain
Perfumery Note: top
Extraction Method: cold pressed / expressed

About: Mandarin is the sweetest of all the essential oils and has restful and soothing effects. Because of this, and its candy-like scent, it is a good choice for helping children sleep. When eaten, mandarins are most often found in Asian salads. Often interchangeable with tangerine oil, mandarin is often chosen because it contains esters.

USES -
Mind: anxiety, restful and soothing, cheering, depression, nerves, stimulating, stress
Body: acne, antidepressant, antiseptic, astringent, digestive, hiccups, insomnia, muscle cramps, oily skin, scars, stomachaches, stretch marks, wrinkles
Spirit: happiness, joy, luck, 2nd chakra (sacral), creativity

Safety Warnings: Phototoxic, do not use before going out in sun. Dilute before using with children.

MARJORAM
Botanical Name: origanum marjorana
Aromatic Profile: sweet, woodsy, spicy, camphorus, herbaceous, slightly fruity
Origin: Turkey, Spain, Cyprus
Perfumery Note: middle
Extraction Method: steam distilled

About: Marjoram is a perennial herb that is sometimes used in place of oregano. It is one of the ingredients used in the culinary herb mixture called *Herbes de Provence*, which is often used on meat dishes and grilling. In ancient Greece it was given to newlyweds to insure good fortune upon their household. The essential oil marjoram is primarily used in massage oil blends due to its effectiveness on sore muscles.

USES -

Mind: aggressive behavior, anxiety, restful and soothing, exhaustion, strengthening, tension
Body: analgesic, antidepressant, anti-inflammatory, antiseptic, antispasmodic, arthritis, bronchitis, carminative, carpal tunnel syndrome, colic, coughing, cramps, drug withdrawal, headaches, insomnia, lowers blood pressure, migraines, muscle relaxant, muscular aches, muscular fatigue, neuralgia, osteoarthritis, rheumatism, sprains
Spirit: inner peace, self-control

Safety Warnings: Avoid during pregnancy or a history of low blood pressure. Not for use on children. May lower sex drive.

MELISSA

Botanical Name: melissa officinalis
Aromatic Profile: herbaceous, green, fresh, slightly lemon-like
Origin: France, Europe
Perfumery Note: top/middle

Extraction Method: steam distilled

About: Melissa is another word for the herb known as lemon balm. It is a perennial herb that is especially good for hay fever due to its anti-histamine properties. The herb, brewed into a tea, is also an effective treatment for herpes flare-ups. Lemon balm is often used as a flavoring in herbal teas and ice cream. Melissa oil is usually very expensive because the plant is high in water and low in essential oil.

USES -
Mind: anxiety, restful and soothing, exhaustion , hysteria, nerves, relaxation, stress, inspirational
Body: antibacterial, antifungal, antiviral, bronchitis, chicken pox, coughing, eczema, flatulence, headaches, indigestion, lowers blood pressure, menstrual cramps, nausea, PMS symptoms, sedative
Spirit: money, success, achievement

Safety Warnings: Dilute well before use on skin. While the herb lemon balm is good for allergies, the intensity of the essential oil may have the opposite effect and trigger allergies.

MYRRH
Botanical Name: commiphora myrrha
Aromatic Profile: woodsy, earthy, warm, exotic
Origin: Ethiopia, Yemen, Somalia
Perfumery Note: base
Extraction Method: steam distilled

About: It is said that myrrh was one of the gifts the Wise Men brought to the baby Jesus. It was also used by the ancient Egyptians as one of the ingredients used in the embalming process. Like frankincense, myrrh is a resin extracted from its tree by wounding the bark and comes out in droplets that become very hard when dry.

USES -

Mind: concentration, focus, memory, stimulates higher thinking

Body: acne, amenorrhea, antibacterial, antifungal, anti-inflammatory, antiseptic, antiviral, athlete's foot, blisters, bronchitis, chapped skin, cuts, dermatitis, diarrhea, emollient, gums, halitosis, itching, ringworm, wounds, wrinkles

Spirit: astral projection, blessing, consecration, meditation, protection, psychic power, spirituality, hex removing

Safety Warnings: Avoid during pregnancy

NEROLI

Botanical Name: citrus aurantium
Aromatic Profile: floral, citrusy, sweet, rich, slightly spicy
Origin: Italy, Morocco
Perfumery Note: middle
Extraction Method: steam distilled

About: Neroli oil comes from the blossoms on the bitter orange tree and its flowers are extremely fragrant. It has been used for centuries as an ingredient in perfumery and is the most common scent used in the fragrance industry. The oil is usually very expensive. It is said to be an effective aphrodisiac.

USES -
Mind: aggressive behavior, aphrodisiac, anxiety, restful and soothing, concentration, creativity, exhaustion, exotic, memory loss, nervous tension, relaxing, self-hypnosis, stress

Body: abrasions, acne, antidepressant, antiseptic, antispasmodic, chapped skin, circulatory stimulant, disinfectant, dry skin, frigidity, insomnia, mature skin, migraines, normalizes blood pressure, scars, sedative, stretch marks, wrinkles

Spirit: attraction, confidence, peace, joy, happiness, satisfaction, love

Safety Warnings: Avoid overuse

NUTMEG
Botanical Name: myristica fragrans
Aromatic Profile: spicy, sweet, woodsy, earthy
Origin: Indonesia, Sumatra
Perfumery Note: middle
Extraction Method: steam distilled

About: Nutmeg is a popular culinary spice and is used in a variety of dishes around the world. In Elizabethan times, it was thought to keep away the plague and was always kept on hand. Used in low doses, it has no adverse effects. However, when used in larger quantities, it can cause dehydration, palpitations, and convulsions.

USES -
Mind: irritability, rejuvenating, stress, inspirational
Body: analgesic, antibiotic, antiseptic, antispasmodic, arthritis, boils, bronchitis, circulatory stimulant, drug withdrawal, fatigue, female infertility, insomnia, menopause, muscle relaxant, muscular aches, neuralgia, normalizes blood pressure, oily skin, osteoarthritis, PMS symptoms, sedative, slow digestion, sprains, strains
Spirit: gambling, luck, money, enhances rituals

Safety Warnings: If used in large quantities, nutmeg oil can be toxic

ORANGE, SWEET
Botanical Name: citrus sinensis
Aromatic Profile: sweet, citrusy, fruity, bright
Origin: China, North America, South America, Spain
Perfumery Note: top
Extraction Method: cold pressed/expressed

About: The orange tree is a flowering evergreen tree that reaches about 30 feet in height. Oranges are the most cultivated tree fruit in the world. It is thought that its origins began in the Asian countries. Orange is one of the most affordable of the essential oils because it is abundant and its essential oil yield is high. Orange oil is found in a variety of cleaning products not only for its fresh smell but for its ability to cut grease.

USES -
Mind: anxiety, restful and soothing, cheering, inspiring, invigorating, lifts the spirit, refreshing,
Body: antidepressant, antiseptic, antispasmodic, astringent, cellulite, colds, constipation, diarrhea, drug withdrawal, flatulence, nervine, normal skin, oily skin, sedative, slow digestion, toning, wrinkles
Spirit: divination, happiness, love, luck, 2nd chakra (sacral)

Safety Warnings: avoid use in the sun. May irritate sensitive skin.

PALMAROSA
Botanical Name: cymbopogon martini
Aromatic Profile: sweet, floral, fruit-like, slightly floral.
Origin: Central America, India, Southeast Asia
Perfumery Note: middle
Extraction Method: steam distilled

About: Palmarosa is a grass that is in the same family as lemongrass. However, it does not have the lemon-like scent associated with its close cousin. Palmarosa is used a great deal in the cosmetics industry, mainly in creams and lotions, because it is said to have skin-repairing qualities. It is also sometimes used as a insect repellent when it comes to the storage of dried beans and some grains.

USES -

Mind: aggressive behavior, anxiety, restful and soothing, creativity, exhaustion, relaxing, self-hypnosis, stress

Body: acne, alopecia, bleeding, circulatory stimulant, convalescence, cuts, dermatitis, dry skin, hair loss, insomnia, muscle relaxant, normal skin, oily skin, PMS symptoms, raises blood pressure, shock, soothing, wounds, wrinkles

Spirit: healing energy, love, acceptance

Safety Warnings: Avoid if a history of high blood pressure.

PATCHOULI

Botanical Name: pogostemon cablin
Aromatic Profile: dark, rich, exotic, earthy, woody
Origin: China, Indonesia, India, Malaysia
Perfumery Note: base
Extraction Method: steam distilled

About: Patchouli is a bushy herb in the mint family that grows about two to three feet tall. However, there are many plants in the mint family that smell nothing like mint – patchouli is one of them. Patchouli is a fixative oil, meaning that if it is used in small amounts it can boost the scent of other oils it is blended with. Patchouli oil has the reputation of being a love-it-or-hate-it oil. Patchouli incense was widely used in the 1960's, which is why it has been given the reputation as the "hippie scent". It was said to mask the scent of marijuana.

USES -
Mind: aphrodisiac, anxiety, restful and soothing, clearing, concentration, exhaustion, fatigue, stress
Body: acne, antibiotic, antidepressant, antifungal, anti-infectious, anti-inflammatory, antiseptic, astringent, athlete's foot, cellulite, chapped skin, dandruff, deodorant, dermatitis, diuretic, dry skin, fixative, mature skin, normal skin, oily skin, wrinkles
Spirit: attraction, banishes negativity, love, luck, money, peace, prosperity, sex

Safety Warnings: Never take internally

PEPPER, BLACK
Botanical Name: piper nigrum
Aromatic Profile: spicy, woodsy, sharp, clean
Origin: India, Indonesia, Madagascar
Perfumery Note: middle
Extraction Method: steam distilled

About: Pepper is probably the most widely used spice, found in nearly every kitchen around the globe. Few know that the plant is actually a vine. It can grow up to thirteen feet tall and usually attaches itself to poles, branches, and other sturdy objects. The plant is native to southern India but is cultivated and grows well in all tropical regions. When it comes to the essential oil, it is mainly used for aching muscles and to improve circulation. However, it should be well-diluted.

USES -

Mind: concentration, energizing, exhaustion, invigorating, revitalizing, warming
Body: anti-inflammatory, arteriosclerosis, arthritis, carminative, circulatory stimulant, colds, detoxifying, diuretic, expectorant, flu, muscle relaxant, muscular aches, muscle cramps, osteoarthritis, raises blood pressure, rheumatism, rheumatoid arthritis, sprains
Spirit: courage, confrontation, perception

Safety Warnings: Possible skin irritant. Avoid if a history of high blood pressure. Dilute well before use on the skin.

PEPPERMINT

Botanical Name: mentha piperita
Aromatic Profile: fresh, cooling, bright, minty
Origin: Europe, North America
Perfumery Note: top
Extraction Method: steam distilled

About: Peppermint is actually a hybrid in the mint family – a cross between spearmint and watermint. It is used to flavor a variety of foods, beverages, and candies. In aromatherapy, it is especially useful for getting rid of a tension headache by simply smelling, in deep breaths, the essential oil.

USES -
Mind: concentration, cooling, exhaustion, invigorating, refreshing, revitalizing, stimulating
Body: ant repellent, antibiotic, anti-inflammatory, antiseptic, antispasmodic, bronchitis, cellulite,

circulatory stimulant, colds, constipation, deodorant,
digestive, disinfectant, fainting, febrifuge, flatulence,
gingivitis, hay fever, headaches, heartburns,
heatstroke, indigestion, jet lag, muscular aches,
nausea, neuralgia, raises blood pressure, rheumatoid
arthritis, sinusitis, tendinitis, abdominal pain, varicose
veins, vomiting, water retention

Spirit: good health, protection, purification,
stimulates the mind

Safety Warnings: avoid during pregnancy or a
history of high blood pressure. Dilute well if used on
skin.

PETITGRAIN

Botanical Name: citrus aurantium
Aromatic Profile: fresh, floral, fruity, slightly woodsy
Origin: Italy, Morocco, South America
Perfumery Note: top
Extraction Method: steam distilled

About: Petitgrain comes from the bitter orange
plant. While neroli comes from the blossom of the
bitter orange and bitter orange oil comes from the
fruit, petitgrain comes from steam distilling the leaves
and twigs of the plant. This is why the oil has a trio of
scents hidden inside: floral, fruity, and woodsy. It is
highly used in the perfume industry.

USES -

Mind: restful and soothing, inspiring, invigorating,
refreshing, relaxing, soothing, stress, inspirational

Body: antibacterial, antidepressant, anti-infectious, anti-inflammatory, antiseptic, antispasmodic, aphrodisiac, deodorant, insomnia, scars, shock
Spirit: attraction, protection, stimulates thought

Safety Warnings: Never take internally

PINE

Botanical Name: pinus sylvestris
Aromatic Profile: balsamic, woodsy, earthy, clean
Origin: Europe, North America, Russia
Perfumery Note: middle
Extraction Method: steam distilled

About: Pines are evergreen trees that have a long life – anywhere between a hundred and a thousand years. There are over one hundred types of pine trees and they are found in many areas of the world, mainly in the Northern Hemisphere. The wood is used for timber and to make some types of furniture as well as chips for animal bedding. The pine needles are often used as landscaping groundcover and at least 20 species of the pine create seed large enough to be eaten, also known as pine nuts.

USES -

Mind: exhaustion, refreshing, rejuvenating, revitalizing, stimulating, strengthening, stress
Body: analgesic, antibacterial, antibiotic, antifungal, antiseptic, antiviral, arthritis, asthma, bronchitis, circulatory stimulant, colds, coughs, decongestant, deodorant, detoxifying, disinfectant, diuretic, eczema,

expectorant, flu, gout, muscular aches, neuralgia, osteoarthritis, psoriasis, raises blood pressure, rheumatism, sinusitis
Spirit: grounding, healing, protection

Safety Warnings: Avoid if a history of high blood pressure or prostate cancer.

RAVENSARA

Botanical Name: ravensara aromatica
Aromatic Profile: medicinal, slightly licorice-like, sweet, dry
Origin: Australia, Madagascar, Tasmania
Perfumery Note: top
Extraction Method: steam distilled

About: Native to Madagascar, Ravensara are evergreen trees that grow well in tropical and subtropical regions. The essential oil is primarily used for medicinal purposes and is said to keep the flu virus away. It is often used in a room spray during the flu season.

USES -
Mind: restful and soothing, clearing, relaxing, soothing
Body: antibacterial, antibiotic, anti-infectious, antiseptic, antiviral, boils, bronchitis, expectorant, influenza, laryngitis, lung infections, pneumonia, sinusitis
Spirit: calm thoughts, clear thinking, problem solving

Safety Warnings: Never take internally

ROSE

Botanical Name: rosa damascena
Aromatic Profile: floral, sweet
Origin: Bulgaria, France
Perfumery Note: middle
Extraction Method: solvent extracted/steam distilled

About: Like jasmine, rose is often solvent extracted because of its delicate petals – this process creates rose absolute.   When the steam distillation process is used, the result is rose otto which is significantly more expensive. Like the flower, rose oil is often associated with love and passion.

USES -

Mind: aphrodisiac, balancing, restful and soothing, cheering, nervous tension, relaxing, stress
Body: acne, Alzheimer's disease, antibacterial, antidepressant, antiseptic, antispasmodic, antiviral, arthritis, astringent, chapped lips, chapped skin, circulatory stimulant, colds, cuts, depression, drug withdrawal, dry skin, eczema, female infertility, frigidity, headaches, insomnia, mature skin, menopause, normal skin, PMS symptoms, raises blood pressure, sedative, shock, wrinkles
Spirit: love, sex, passion

Safety Warnings: Avoid during pregnancy or a history of high blood pressure

ROSEMARY

Botanical Name: rosmarinus officinalis
Aromatic Profile: fresh, herbaceous, clean, hint of sweetness
Origin: France, Spain, Mediterranean
Perfumery Note: middle
Extraction Method: steam distilled

About: Rosemary is a perennial herb with needle like leaves and purple flowers. The essential oil content is high in rosemary, evident when one runs their hand along a stem of leaves.   It is widely used in cooking to flavor meats and is an excellent ingredient in hair care products.

USES -
Mind: concentration, fatigue, grief, inspiring, invigorating, memory loss, nervous tension, stimulating
Body: alopecia, analgesic, antidepressant, anti-inflammatory, antiseptic, antispasmodic, antiviral, arthritis, asthma, bronchitis, bruises, circulatory stimulant, colds, constipation, cramps, cystitis, dandruff, decongestant, digestive, disinfectant, dry skin, flu, gout, hair loss, hangovers, headaches, immune system, lice, lower abdominal pain, lumbago, moth repellent, muscular aches, osteoporosis, raises blood pressure, rheumatism, rheumatoid arthritis, sinusitis, sprains, swelling, tendinitis
Spirit: nostalgia, protection, yoga, 4th chakra (heart), sixth chakra

Safety Warnings: Avoid during pregnancy or a history of epilepsy or high blood pressure.

SANDALWOOD

Botanical Name: santalum album
Aromatic Profile: perfume-like, sweet, woodsy, rich
Origin: India, Australia, Tasmania
Perfumery Note: base
Extraction Method: steam distilled

About: Sandalwood has been used for centuries for use in spiritual, religious, and meditation practices and ceremonies. Its fragrance can last for many years in the wood, long after the tree has been cut down. Much used in the perfume industry, it is also used as an aphrodisiac.

USES -

Mind: aphrodisiac, calming, centering, exhaustion, grounding, relaxing, stress
Body: acne, antifungal, anti-inflammatory, antiseptic, antispasmodic, antiviral, astringent, carminative, chapped skin, coughs, cystitis, diarrhea, diuretic, drug withdrawal, dry hair, dry skin, emollient, hair, immunity stimulant, insomnia, normal skin, sedative, skin conditioner, wrinkles
Spirit: anointing, attraction, blessing, consecration, love, meditation, protection, purification, 2nd chakra (sacral), spirituality

Safety Warnings: Never take sandalwood internally.

SPEARMINT

Botanical Name: mentha spicata
Aromatic Profile: minty, sweet, fresh, slightly fruity
Origin: China, Europe, North America
Perfumery Note: top
Extraction Method: steam distilled

About: Spearmint is a species of mint that is native to Asia and Europe. It is known as an invasive plant, sending shoots underground. Besides being used in candies and toothpaste, it is also found in beverages such as mint julep and the mojito. Spearmint is especially good for covering up unwanted smells and is a pleasing scent.   Essential oil of spearmint is often used as a replacement for those who find the scent of peppermint too strong.

USES -

Mind: energizing, refreshing, stimulating, inspirational
Body: ant repellent, antiseptic, asthma, deodorant, exhaustion, fever, flatulence, indigestion, morning sickness, moth repellent, mouse repellent, nausea, nervine, soothing agent, stomachaches, vertigo
Spirit: comfort, protection, security

Safety Warnings: Possible mucous membrane irritation

TANGERINE

Botanical Name: citrus reticulata
Aromatic Profile: citrusy, fruity, tangy, sweet, fresh

Origin: China, Morocco, South America, North America
Perfumery Note: top
Extraction Method: cold pressed/expressed

About: Tangerines are a citrus fruit related to the mandarin orange. They are smaller in size than regular oranges and usually much sweeter. The name was derived from Tangiers (Morocco), the port in which it was first exported to parts of Europe. Tangerine has a restful and soothing effect and works well when blended with other oils for the same purpose such as lavender.

USES -

Mind: restful and soothing, cheering, relaxing, soothing, stress, inspirational
Body: antidepressant, antiseptic, antispasmodic, astringent, cellulite, dandruff, insomnia, lymphatic cleanser, muscle relaxant, oily skin, sedative, stretch marks
Spirit: enhances magical work, purification

Safety Warnings: Possibly phototoxic – avoid overuse in the sun

TEA TREE

Botanical Name: melaleuca alternifolia
Aromatic Profile: fresh, medicinal, herbaceous, clean, green
Origin: Australia, China
Perfumery Note: middle

Extraction Method: steam distilled

About: The indigenous people of Australia have known about the healing properties of tea tree for thousands of years. The leaves were often soaked to apply poultices to wounds or were inhaled for respiratory infections. Tea tree has shown to be effective in treating athlete's foot and other fungus and yeast infections. It is found in many products that treat acne. During World War II, Australian soldiers carried tea tree oil in their first aid kits.

USES -
Mind: cleansing, cooling, energizing, stimulating, inspirational
Body: abrasions, abscesses, acne, antibacterial, antifungal, anti-infectious, anti-inflammatory, antiseptic, antiviral, athlete's foot, blisters, boils, bronchitis, candida, catarrh, cold sores, colds, cuts, ear infections, fevers, flu, herpes, insect bites, jock itch, mumps, pneumonia, ringworm, shock, sinusitis, sunburns, thrush, toothaches, vaginal infections, warts, wounds, yeast infections
Spirit: cleanses negativity, purification

Safety Warnings: Not for internal use.

YLANG YLANG
Botanical Name: cananga odorata
Aromatic Profile: floral, sweet, earthy
Origin: Indonesia, Madagascar
Perfumery Note: middle/base

Extraction Method: steam distilled

About: The tree grows extremely fast and can reach forty feet in height. It has been prized for centuries for its powerful fragrance and its aphrodisiac properties. The people of Indonesia would spread ylang-ylang flowers across the marital bed of a newlywed couple. It is highly used in the perfume industry and is one of the ingredients in Chanel No 5.

USES -
Mind: aggression, aphrodisiac, anxiety, balancing, restful and soothing, cooling, euphoric, relaxing
Body: antidepressant, antiseptic, disinfectant, lowers blood pressure, normal skin, oily skin, sedative, shock
Spirit: love, lust, sex, peace

Safety Warnings: Avoid if a history of low blood pressure

CLOSING

I hope this book has given you a clear understanding about essential oils and aromatherapy. We have covered the history of aromatherapy, how to use the oils, the chemistry of essential oils, how to create a balanced blend, how essential oils are made, the carrier oils used in blends, scent notes, a few questionable aspects of the industry, recipes to get you started, and a complete encyclopedia of the top fifty-five oils.

When you begin your adventure into using essential oils, start on a small scale. If there is an oil you have never tried and can't sample it locally, order the smallest bottle available and work up to larger sizes later. This way you can afford to build your supply of oils with a wider variety. Also, smaller amounts let you "test out" different suppliers until you find the one that is best suited to you and offers the quality you are looking for.

Creating your own blends for beauty, health, and spiritual needs is a rewarding experience and can quickly become addicting. Before you know it, you'll be taking more hot baths, trading massages with your significant-other, making your own perfume, and mixing up bags of aromatherapy bath salts for holiday gifts. If nothing else, your house is going to smell amazing.

RESOURCES

AROMAGREGORY CREATIVE INC.
essential oils, handmade soaps, bulk wholesale soap, classes
www.aromagregory.com

NAHA – National Association of Holistic Aromatherapy
leading aromatherapy association in United States
www.naha.org

CFA – Canadian Federation of Aromatherapy
promoting education and true aromatherapy standards for Canada
www.cfacanada.com

ALLIANCE OF INTERNATIONAL AROMATHERAPISTS
international member-based organization promoting true
aromatherapy
www.alliance-aromatherapists.org

AROMAWEB
online resource for all things aromatherapy + business listings
www.aromaweb.com

LIBERTY NATURAL
bulk essential oils and aromatherapy supplies
www.libertynatural.com

INTERNATIONAL CERTIFIED AROMATHERAPY INSTITUTE
aromatherapy education, certification – Marlene Mitchell, director
– Canada
www.aromatherapyinstitute.com

ATLANTIC INSTITUTE OF AROMATHERAPY
aromatherapy education, certification – Tampa, Florida
www.atlanticinstitute.com

ABOUT THE AUTHOR

Gregory Lee White is a writer and a certified clinical aromatherapist. He lives in Nashville, Tennessee. His soap company is aromagregory.com.
Author website: www.gregoryleewhite.com

Made in the USA
Charleston, SC
16 September 2015